The Young Athlete's Handbook

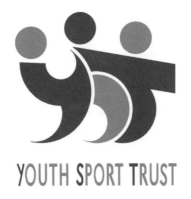

YOUTH SPORT TRUST

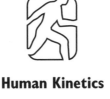

Human Kinetics

Library of Congress Cataloging-in-Publication Data

Youth Sport Trust (Great Britain)
    The young athlete's handbook / Youth Sport Trust ; [written by Penny Crisfield ... et al.].
        p. cm.
    ISBN 0-7360-3712-8
    1. Athletes--Training of--Great Britain--Handbooks, manuals, etc. 2. Physical fitness
for youth--Great Britain--Handbooks, manuals, etc.   I. Crisfield, Penny.   II. Title.

    GV711.5 .Y68   2001
    613.7'11--dc21   00-054240

ISBN: 0-7360-3712-8

This book is a revised edition of *Planning for Success: Performer's Diary,* published in 1999 by the Institute of Youth Sport at Loughborough University.

Writers: Penny Crisfield, Chris Earle, Chris Harwood, Lisa Piearce, Sarah Rowell and Mark Simpson; **Developmental Editors**: Diane Evans and Laura Hambly; **Assistant Editor**: Stephan Seyfert; **Copyeditor**: Barbara Field; **Proofreader**: Myla Smith; **Permission Manager**: Toni Harte; **Graphic Designer**: Nancy Rasmus; **Graphic Artist**: Sandra Meier; **Photo Editor**: Clark Brooks; **Cover Designer**: Keith Blomberg; **Photographer (cover)**: Tom Roberts; **Photographer (interior)**: Tom Roberts, unless otherwise noted; **Illustrator**: Tom Roberts; **Printer**: United Graphics

Human Kinetics books are available at special discounts for bulk purchase. Special editions or book excerpts can also be created to specification. For details, contact the Special Sales Manager at Human Kinetics.

Printed in the United States of America   10   9   8   7   6   5   4   3   2   1

Human Kinetics
Web site: www.humankinetics.com

United States: Human Kinetics
P.O. Box 5076, Champaign, IL 61825-5076
800-747-4457
e-mail: humank@hkusa.com

Canada: Human Kinetics
475 Devonshire Road Unit 100
Windsor, ON N8Y 2L5
800-465-7301 (in Canada only)
e-mail: hkcan@mnsi.net

Europe: Human Kinetics
Units C2/C3 Wira Business Park
West Park Ring Road
Leeds LS16 6EB, United Kingdom
+44 (0) 113 278 1708

e-mail: humank@hkeurope.com

Australia: Human Kinetics
57A Price Avenue, Lower Mitcham
South Australia 5062
08 8277 1555
e-mail: liahka@senet.com.au

New Zealand: Human Kinetics
P.O. Box 105-231, Auckland Central
09-523-3462
e-mail: hkp@ihug.co.nz

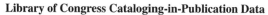

The Youth Sport Trust would like to thank all those who assisted in the writing, consulting and publishing of this book. It would not have been possible without key contributions from Jonny Nye and Dave Williams in the sports marketing department at Nike UK and staff members at both UK Sport and the British Olympic Association.

CONTENTS

iv

FOREWORD

Congratulations for getting this far in your chosen sport. Well done for spending time training when you could have been doing other activities, for balancing all the commitments that a young person has these days and for having those special characteristics that give you the potential to be a great performer one day.

Many of you may feel you have already come a long way in your sport and have committed a great deal of time, money, training and effort. You may already compete at quite a high level and spend a considerable amount of time training and practising the sport you love. I want you to look at this as the beginning. I want you to start taking more responsibility for your own progress, and this book will help you. It will help you learn what elite athletes do to help them gain the most from their training: how they work with their coach, how they build specific fitness plans for their sport, how they eat and how they ensure their minds are as fit as their bodies. It will help you be the best you can.

You may already have a great team trying to help you: your parent or guardian, coach, teacher, physiotherapist or doctor and friends. They are all very important to your success and happiness. However, you can also begin to take more responsibility for your own progress. Who better? You are the only one who really knows how much you can do and how successful you want to be.

I hope you find this book helpful and start to use your own diary to monitor your progress along the path to success. Good luck with your sporting future.

With very best wishes,

Steve Cram

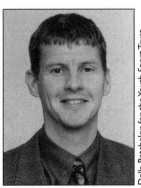

Steve Cram competed in the golden era of British middle-distance running and became world champion in 1983. In 1985, he claimed world records in the mile, the 1,500 metres, and the 2,000 metres, all in 19 days. A commentator and presenter for BBC sport and chairman of the English Institute of Sport, Steve is now passing on his knowledge and enthusiasm to a new generation of athletes.

HOW TO USE THIS BOOK

The Young Athlete's Handbook has been written to help you and other talented young sportspersons become the very best athletes you can. It will help you enjoy training and become a more successful athlete, prepared for the sporting and other challenges that lie ahead. It will help you get the most from your training but, at the same time, keep your sport balanced with other important aspects of your life, including friends, family, school and other hobbies. It provides many helpful tips on key issues such as fitness, diet, injury, mental skills and nutrition, as well as useful information on topics such as travel and drug testing, that you can use for reference as needed. To provide you with the very best information, a number of top organisations and individuals have been involved: sport scientists from Loughborough University, experts from the British Olympic Association and staff from UK Sport.

This book is not intended as a substitute for a good coach, supportive parent or guardian or your physiotherapist. It has been written to help you better understand everything that is involved in becoming a successful athlete and to enable you to take more responsibility for your own progress. You are strongly encouraged to share the information with all those who work with you, and at various times, you are specifically reminded to discuss certain topics with your coach, teacher or parent or guardian.

You should also use this book in conjunction with a training diary to help you plan and record your progress. In the last chapter, you will find a sample diary to help you put your new skills and knowledge into good training practice. You can choose to use these pages as your own training diary or convert your current personal diary into a training diary. Whatever diary you use, make sure it suits you (and your sport) and is easy and fun to use.

The Young Athlete's Handbook is divided into four parts. Each part is divided into chapters containing useful information and some simple tasks to help you work out how this information can make a difference in your sport. When reading the book for the first time, it is a good idea to complete all the chapters in order. After that, however, you might prefer to dip into the chapters when they seem relevant or you need them. The first chapter helps you analyse the unique demands and specific training requirements of your sport. It shows you how to identify your strengths and weaknesses and decide where you need the most work. Chapter 2 helps you get the most from your training but, at the same time, achieve a balanced lifestyle so that sport does not dominate every aspect of your life.

In Part II, Improving Mind and Body, you will find chapters on four factors that strongly influence your sporting success: fitness, diet, mental skills and sport injuries. Here you will find more useful tips you can put into practice. You will be able to identify which fitness components (endurance, speed, strength, flexibility) are most important for you and how best to develop them, ways to ensure that you eat the right foods to give you plenty of energy for training, ideas on how to improve your concentration and reminders on how to stay healthy and avoid injuries.

Part III, Getting Serious, provides some key information that you will inevitably need at some point: tips on training and competing abroad and information on drugs and dope testing.

In the final part, Planning for Success, you start to do some real planning for the forthcoming season. It shows you how to develop your own training diary, how to set goals and plan your training schedules and ways to log your progress on the exciting pathway to your sporting success.

Enjoy using this handbook, and good luck with your sport.

Starting to Plan

It is important to develop good training habits now that can last you the whole of your sporting career. Missing the odd training session does not matter; it's the training consistency over months and years that is important.

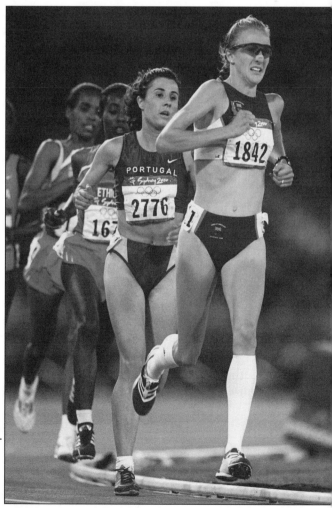

© EMPICS/Simpson

Every sport is different. Some are very technical (gymnastics, javelin and fencing, for example). Others, including games such as football and hockey, are also very tactical. Some make enormous demands on fitness (e.g., triathlons, distance running and swimming), whereas in others (e.g., shooting and the short sprint events), the mental side is more important. Therefore, the first step in planning for your success is to identify the unique demands of your sport so you can determine your specific training requirements. Chapter 1 (Knowing Your Sport and Yourself) will help you do this by showing you how to analyse top performers in your sport to identify the attributes (skills, knowledge, attitudes) that seem to be important for success. Through a process called 'performance profiling', you will then be able to identify your own strengths and weaknesses and decide where you need to do the most work. You will have further opportunities to use the profiling in the last chapter, where you can combine all the information you have gleaned and plan for your success.

Chapter 2 (Training Smarter) helps you get the most from your training but, at the same time, achieve a balanced lifestyle so that sport does not dominate every aspect of your life. This balance is important, given that many talented athletes fail to reach their potential because they are either injured (often as a result of poor training schedules) or become burned out. They lose their motivation to train and even to compete. They have had enough and want to do other things with their lives. When you train, therefore, it is vital to ensure you are gaining the most from it. In this book, it is called training smart; not necessarily advocating more training, but training in a more effective way and with greater quality. It is also essential to find time for all the other things that are important to you and your future. This not only includes school, career, holidays and other hobbies and interests, but also spending time with those who make up *Team You*, meaning all the people who help you to be successful (such as your coach, family, friends, teachers and medical support staff). This chapter helps you to prioritise and then fit time into your weekly schedule for everything that is important to you.

Once you have worked through these chapters, you can start to identify the other topics in this book that will make a real difference in your sport performance. Perhaps you want to know more about nutrition or how to develop mental skills. You will be able to find out how to work on these aspects of your performance and decide exactly what training plan will make the greatest difference. Remember, it is important to discuss your ideas regularly with *Team You*, especially your coach and your parent or guardian.

Knowing Your Sport and Yourself

How well do you know yourself and your sport? Every sport and every athlete is different, so before you can plan your way to sporting success, you must first analyse exactly what it takes to be an elite athlete in your sport. This means you look closely at your sport to identify its essential requirements: the physical requirements such as speed or endurance; the psychological demands such as commitment and concentration; and the technical and tactical requirements (e.g., the abilities to throw and catch, play a zone defence, perform a range of tumbling skills or run over a flight of hurdles). Next you identify all the attributes (the skills, knowledge and attitudes) that seem to describe the outstanding and successful athletes in your sport. Finally, you use a profiling technique to rate yourself on all these attributes so you know your strengths and areas you need to work particularly hard to improve. This chapter is divided into two sections:

1. Analysing your sport
2. Profiling yourself

Analysing Your Sport

The type and amount of training you do depends not only on your ambitions, but on the specific requirements of your sport. Most sports make demands in the following performance areas:

- Physical – the need for endurance, strength, speed, power and flexibility, and therefore proper diet and nutrition
- Technical – the ability to execute specific actions or skills
- Tactical – the ability to make decisions on how to maximise your success and reduce the effectiveness of the opposition
- Mental – the need for mental toughness: concentration, commitment, control and confidence

Specific Requirements of Your Sport

All of the above performance areas make demands on your lifestyle; however, the relative importance of each of them will depend on the specific require-

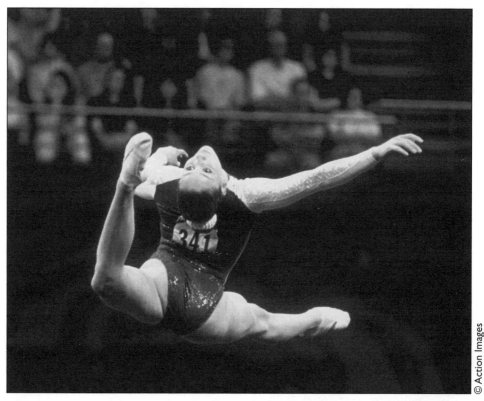

Gymnasts focus on power, flexibility and skills training because of the high physical and technical demands of their sport.

ments of your sport at your performance level. For example, distance running and swimming make significant physical demands (particularly for endurance) and mental demands for commitment or effort; gymnastics requires power and flexibility, as well as strong technical skills; football and hockey make particularly strong tactical demands. The relative priorities might also vary for different performance levels. For example, for young hockey players, the technical requirements might be deemed more important than the physical demands; however, with senior national players, the opposite might be true. Before you start to plan your training, therefore, the first step must be to analyse the specific requirements of your sport at your performance level so that you can tailor your training appropriately. Tasks 1 and 2 will help you do this.

> The first step in planning for success is to analyse the unique requirements of your sport. Then you plan your training for working on the areas that are most important.

Task 1   Rating Areas of Importance in Your Sport

First, rate the relative importance of each area for you in your sport. Some examples are provided in the shaded panels, and you might want to check your ideas with your coach, teacher or parent or guardian.

Example from junior rugby

	Unimportant				Very important
Physical/fitness	1	2	③	4	5
Technical	1	2	3	4	⑤
Tactical	1	2	3	④	5
Mental	1	2	③	4	5

Example from senior swimming (sprint events)

	Unimportant				Very important
Physical/fitness	1	2	3	④	5
Technical	1	2	3	4	⑤
Tactical	①	2	3	4	5
Mental	1	2	③	4	5

(continued)

Task 1 *(continued)*

	Unimportant				Very important
Physical/fitness	1	2	3	4	5
Technical	1	2	3	4	5
Tactical	1	2	3	4	5
Mental	1	2	3	4	5

Now try answering the following questions in Task 2 to analyse your sport in more detail.

Task 2 Analysing Your Sport in Detail

In terms of the fitness demands, do you have to:

keep moving actively for more than 2-3 min. at a time without a break (e.g., hockey, football, distance running/swimming)?	Y/N	If yes, aerobic endurance is a requirement.
carry out repeated bouts of harder exercise, which last up to a minute (e.g., sprinting in many sports, high/long jump)?	Y/N	If yes, anaerobic (speed) endurance is a requirement.
move as fast as possible at times (e.g., netball, fencing, sprinting)?	Y/N	If yes, speed is a requirement.
change direction at speed (e.g., netball, tennis)?	Y/N	If yes, speed agility is important.
make strong, fast movements such as throwing, jumping or lifting (e.g., tennis, cricket, basketball, rugby)?	Y/N	If yes, power is a requirement.
make repeated strong fast movements such as kicking or hitting without a break (e.g., tennis, squash)?	Y/N	If yes, muscular endurance is a requirement.
move or resist heavy objects or other performers (e.g., rugby, throwing events)?	Y/N	If yes, strength is a requirement.

make sudden or extreme movements such as lunging or twisting, or do you need a large range of movement (e.g., gymnastics, netball, rugby)?	Y/N	If yes, flexibility is a requirement.

In terms of the technical and tactical demands, do you have to:

execute techniques in a specified way (e.g., gymnastics, ice skating, diving)?	Y/N	If yes, there is a high technical demand.
repeatedly execute techniques in an efficient way (e.g., cycling, rowing, swimming)?	Y/N	If yes, the development of an efficient technique is important.
execute techniques to achieve a particular purpose (e.g., make a successful pass, score a goal), rather than conform to a specified movement pattern?	Y/N	If yes, technical demand may be less important than tactical.
make a lot of quick decisions (e.g., about when, how or where to move, pass or hit)?	Y/N	If yes, there is a high tactical demand.

In terms of the mental demands:

do you have to concentrate for long periods (e.g., netball, swimming, rugby)?	Y/N	If yes, maintaining concentration is important.
do you have to concentrate, then switch off, then concentrate again (e.g., golf, archery, gymnastics)?	Y/N	If yes, the ability to refocus is important.
do you have to endure significant levels of fatigue, pain or discomfort (e.g., distance events)?	Y/N	If yes, commitment and determination are important.
do you have to train hard for long periods most days (e.g., swimming, distance running)?	Y/N	If yes, training commitment is important.
do you have to work in a team (e.g., football, rowing)?	Y/N	If yes, teamwork and interaction are important.

(continued)

Task 2 *(continued)*

do you perform in the same playing area as the opposition (e.g., netball, hockey)?	Y/N	If yes, emotional and physical control may be important.
is there physical contact (e.g., rugby)?	Y/N	If yes, emotional and physical control will be important.
does the opposition's performance directly affect your ability to perform (e.g., tennis)?	Y/N	If yes, emotional control and self-confidence may be important.
does the official have an effect on your performance during the event (e.g., football, basketball)?	Y/N	If yes, emotional control may be important.

Once you have completed Task 2, you may want to discuss your answers with your coach, teacher or parent or guardian. You may also need to go back and alter your responses in Task 1. You will need to look back at Task 2 at various times as you work through the book.

Annual Training Programme

Your sport also makes different demands on you at different times of the year. There will be times when you are heavily involved in competitions, times when you are training hard and other times when you can and should take a break from your sport. Sports sometimes use different terms to describe these phases, but the following should be easily applied:

- Transition or recovery phase – the time following all the competitions when you have a complete break from your sport and training. It might last a few weeks or even a couple of months.
- Preseason preparation – the time when you return to training and before any competitions start. It's the time to work on general fitness, on improving techniques and on developing mental skills.
- Early-season preparation – the time when training starts to increase in intensity and become more specific. Typically, although there might be some competitions, the focus is still on preparing for the more important competitions to come later in the season.
- Competition phase – the time when the focus is very much on competing, when you have the most important competitions and want to perform at your very best.

The next task will help you work out when these phases occur in your sport. Afterwards, you may want to check your plan with your coach, teacher or parent or guardian.

Task 3   Mapping Out the Four Training Phases

Use the following year planner to map out the four phases in your annual programme for your sport. You might want to start by plotting the most important competitions and identifying the competition phase; then work backwards and identify the early-season, preseason and transition phases. Look at the example from netball and then try to complete your own (top two rows only for now).

Example Annual Programme for a Junior Netball Club

	Jan.	Feb.	Mar.	Apr.	May	June	July	Aug.	Sep.	Oct.	Nov.	Dec.
Phases	Competition phase				Recovery phase		Preseason phase		Early-season phase			
Sport	League matches Schools Junior Tourn. County champs.											

	Jan.	Feb.	Mar.	Apr.	May	June	July	Aug.	Sep.	Oct.	Nov.	Dec.
Phases												
Sport												
School												
Social												
Other												

You will have a chance to come back and complete Task 3 later on. The ideal time to plan your annual programme is during the recovery phase before the preseason training. However, if you are already in the preseason or early-season phase, it is still worth mapping out your season in this way.

Profiling Yourself

What are your strengths? How can you strengthen your weaknesses? Many elite athletes now use profiling to help them identify their strengths and weaknesses and prioritise their training. It's a simple process in which you first identify what you feel are the most important attributes (knowledge, skills and attitude) needed to become an elite performer. You then rate yourself on how much you feel you possess each attribute right now. This helps you decide on which areas you need to work to become a better performer and so achieve your full potential.

For example, attributes of an elite athlete might include

- *knowledge* of the rules, about equipment, tactics, diet and fitness;
- *skills* such as technical skills, concentration and planning; and
- *attitude*, such as commitment, honesty and teamwork.

Self-profiling is valuable because it requires self-reflection and analysis, and these are important qualities of high achievers. Self-profiling encourages you to

- be aware of your attributes and weaknesses in all aspects of sport performance (physical, mental, technical, tactical, diet), as well as in other aspects of your life (school, lifestyle management).
- compare your profile with the very best in your sport.
- discuss your profile with your coach (or teacher or parent or guardian) and identify where you agree and disagree; this helps to build a healthy and open relationship.
- identify areas to work on that you believe will have the greatest impact on your performance.
- take responsibility and focus your training effort and motivation by setting goals.
- monitor your progress by comparing recent profiles with previous ones.
- train smarter so you focus on important areas and are motivated by seeing the improvements you are making.

The more aware you make yourself of your strengths and weaknesses, the clearer the pathway to success will be.

To complete your first profile, you will need to complete the following blank profile form. You may want to look at the example of the squash player's profile on page 13 before you start.

Task 4 Self-Profiling Exercise

Think of the ideal athlete in your sport. It may help to think of a few elite athletes who you admire. In the spaces below, write down all the attributes (skills, knowledge, attitudes) that are important for success. Remember to include all aspects of performance (technical, tactical, mental and physical, in both training and competition), as well as any aspects of their lifestyles with which you are familiar. If helpful, you may wish to look back at your answers to the questions in Task 2 or ask your coach, teacher or parent or guardian for help:

Knowledge: _____

_____

_____

_____

Skills: _____

_____

_____

_____

Attitude: _____

_____

_____

_____

Lifestyle: _____

_____

_____

_____

(continued)

Task 4 *(continued)*

Now select 10 attributes you feel are the most important for success in your sport and write them in the following left-hand column. Across from each attribute, in the centre column, briefly explain what you mean. Then rate yourself honestly (this should be your opinion; no guidance from your coach, teacher or anyone else) on the 10-point scale (1 = very poor and 10 = could not be better). When rating yourself, think of the athlete you want to become (i.e., few, if any, 10s); leave room for improvement.

Attributes	Description	Rating
1.		1 2 3 4 5 6 7 8 9 10
2.		1 2 3 4 5 6 7 8 9 10
3.		1 2 3 4 5 6 7 8 9 10
4.		1 2 3 4 5 6 7 8 9 10
5.		1 2 3 4 5 6 7 8 9 10
6.		1 2 3 4 5 6 7 8 9 10
7.		1 2 3 4 5 6 7 8 9 10
8.		1 2 3 4 5 6 7 8 9 10
9.		1 2 3 4 5 6 7 8 9 10
10.		1 2 3 4 5 6 7 8 9 10

Sample Profile for a Female Squash Player

Attributes	Description	Rating
1. Speed/agility	Get around court fast, change direction at speed	1 2 3 4 5 ⑥ 7 8 9 10
2. Tightness of length	Keep ball to good length all the time	1 2 3 4 ⑤ 6 7 8 9 10
3. Concentration on every point	Maintain focus on the present	1 2 3 4 5 6 ⑦ 8 9 10
4. Aggressive attitude	Determined, no sympathy for opponent	1 2 3 4 5 ⑥ 7 8 9 10
5. Pre-match preparation	Thorough, clear goals and strategies	1 2 3 4 5 6 ⑦ 8 9 10
6. Fast recovery to the T	Work hard throughout, effort to get to the T always	1 2 3 4 ⑤ 6 7 8 9 10
7. Accurate volleys from front	Look for volleys and not waste any	1 2 3 ④ 5 6 7 8 9 10
8. Good stamina, no fatigue	Able to keep going throughout, no letup	1 2 3 4 5 6 ⑦ 8 9 10
9. Determined when behind	Gutsy, never say die	1 2 3 4 5 6 ⑦ 8 9 10
10. Composure and emotional control	Show no emotion, clear headed	1 2 3 4 ⑤ 6 7 8 9 10

In the example profile, the squash player recognises that compared with an elite player, her weakest technical area is her volleys from the front court. Figure 1.1 takes the squash player's current ratings from Task 4 and compares them to her desired ratings, or where she wants to be by the end of the season.

These numbers are then recorded on a circular profile chart as shown in figure 1.1. This helps identify the areas where the most improvement is needed. Use these examples to help create your own circular profile in Task 5.

Attribute	Current rating	Desired rating
Speed/agility	6	7
Tightness of length	5	7
Concentration on every point	7	9
Aggressive attitude	6	6
Pre-match preparation	7	9
Fast recovery to the T	5	7
Accurate volleys from the front court	4	6
High levels of stamina/no fatigue	7	8
Determination when behind	7	9
Composure and emotional control	5	8

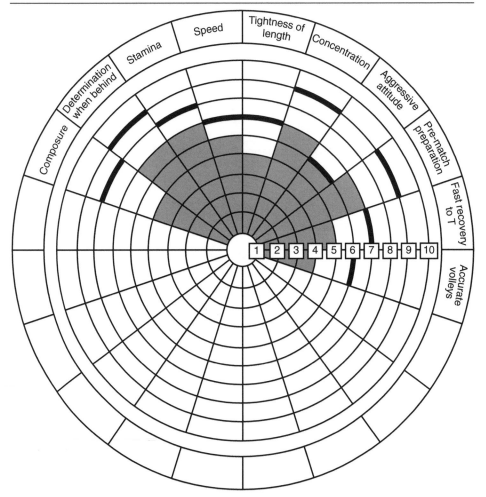

Figure 1.1   Sample circular profile for a female squash player. The shaded areas represent current scores and the bold lines indicate desired ratings.

Task 5   Creating a Profile Chart

You can now record your attributes and scores on the following circular profile chart. Write the attributes around the outside perimeter (see the squash player's example profile) and then shade in your current rating (if you gave yourself a 4, shade in the segment from the centre up to the 4 ring).

It should now be easy to analyse your profile and look at your relative strengths and weaknesses.

Next decide where you would like to be on each attribute by the end of the season (or after 12 months). Be realistic (you can't expect to make big differences on every one; notice that in the previous example, the squash player is typically looking for an improvement of about 1 or 2), but give yourself a challenge. You may want to prioritise and go for a bigger improvement on those attributes you feel

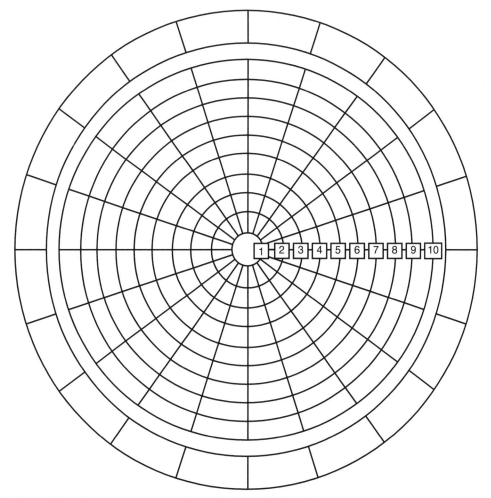

Figure 1.2   Create your own circular profile using this blank form.

(continued)

Task 5 *(continued)*

would have a significant positive impact on your performance (the squash player is striving for a 3 rating improvement on emotional control).

Mark the segment on the score you want to attain (e.g., the squash player is looking to move from a rating of 6 to 7 on speed/agility).

This exercise has helped you learn how to self-profile. It has also given you a first stab at analysing your own strengths and weaknesses against the attributes you believe describe an excellent athlete in your sport and determining a target rating for each attribute for the season. You now need to talk to your coach about which are the priorities and specifically how you should go about achieving them (the section on goal setting and action planning in chapter 5 on page 83 will help you). However, as you work through other chapters in this book, you may find you want to change some of the attributes or analyse them still further. For this reason, you are advised to set aside this profile for now and come back to it later in chapter 9.

Key Points

- Know yourself and your sport. This will help you improve your performance.
- Analyse your sport and find its specific requirements.
- Work out the different demands your sport makes at different times of the year and tailor your training accordingly.
- Profile yourself to find out your strengths and weaknesses.

CHAPTER 2

Training Smarter

Once you know what is required to be a successful athlete in your sport, you can begin to look at how you can organise your life so that you have time for all the things that matter – your sport, your friends, your family, your school life and so on. In this chapter, you will be encouraged to maintain a balance between your sporting life and the rest of your life, for this will help you achieve success and fulfilment in every aspect of your life. Keeping sport important but in harmony with everything else will greatly improve your chances of achieving your sporting potential. You will also receive some basic advice on training effectively – not simply training more but training smarter. This means that when you do commit time to training, it is high quality and purposeful and will make a significant difference to your sporting success.

This chapter is divided into three sections:

1. Maintaining a balanced lifestyle
2. Designing effective training sessions
3. Warming up and cooling down

Maintaining a Balanced Lifestyle

Does sport take over your life? Even the most elite performers should not devote their entire lives to training and competing. Although your sport is important, it should also be part of a balanced lifestyle. Your sport should not take over your life, and you should still have time for other hobbies, family, friends and, of course, your schoolwork. Balancing all these competing demands on your time is difficult; however, careful planning and good communication will help make it possible.

Maintaining this balance and having fun is as important as developing a sporting attitude that helps you maximise the hard physical, mental and technical training you need to ensure you meet your sporting potential. There will obviously be times when you spend more time on one area of your life than another. For example,

- sport will be a high priority in the buildup to a major competition,
- school will be the top priority during exam time, and
- your family or friends are important when on holiday or on special occasions such as Christmas.

Even during these times, it is unlikely you will be concentrating on one area to the exclusion of all else; even full-time professional performers do not train all day every day.

Team You

Team You is important to your success and enjoyment in your sport and your life in general. This team may be made up of all sorts of people with differing roles and responsibilities. It is likely to include your parent or guardian, coach, teacher, friends and perhaps other support staff such as a physiotherapist, doctor or sport scientist – anyone who in any way helps you with your sport and with keeping your life in balance. Once you have identified *Team You*, it is important that you communicate with them all regularly to share your goals and your progress. It is also important that they communicate regularly with each other to ensure they are working well together.

Task 6 will help set up *Team You* effectively and ensure it works well.

Task 6   Identifying *Team You*

Write down the names of all the people who are currently part of *Team You* and add the names of anyone who you feel could be valuable to have in your team:

Name	Title (e.g., coach, father, physiologist)	Role (how each might help you)

Consider the following questions:

Is each team member aware of your goals and dreams?

Does everyone know how you are trying to reach those goals?

Do they know their roles in helping you?

Are they doing everything they can to help you?

Do you talk to your team members regularly?

Write down one action you will now take to help *Team You* work better for you:

School

School and education are important. Very few performers are lucky enough to become full-time athletes in their sport. Fewer still are able to make a living at their sport. Most athletes who become full time do so only for a short time. Therefore, it is vital that you not neglect your studies at this stage. You can always take time out after your A-levels or university course to concentrate on your sport, but getting your GCSEs and A-levels first is important.

You may find that trying to fit in school, homework, training and competition is difficult and leaves little time for anything else. If this happens, talk to your coach and teacher (and perhaps your parent or guardian as well). If they know your time pressures, they can help you overcome them. For example,

- let your coach know when you have important exams or assignments coming up and need more study time so your training programme can be adjusted accordingly;
- tell your teacher when you have a major competition coming up and will be training hard or attending training camps away; and
- make sure your parent or guardian knows the dates of important training camps and competitions well in advance.

Don't try to struggle along alone; this will only cause you greater stress and is likely to lead to poorer performances, both sporting and academic.

Family

Never forget your family. It is sometimes easy to take for granted those who wash your dirty kit, take you to training and competitions, cook your meals, buy your equipment, cheer for you, celebrate with you when you do well and are there for you when things don't go to plan. Always try to be appreciative of the effort they put in to supporting you, even though this can be difficult if you are tired and have not done as well as you had hoped.

Friends

Everyone needs friends, both in and outside sport. Friends can be part of *Team You*. They can help you overcome your disappointments as well as share in your successes. It is often easier to have friends who compete in the same sport as you. Not only do they have a common interest, but you will likely spend a lot of time with them training and competing. Although it is more difficult to make and keep friendships with people outside your sport, such friendships are also important. It often takes extra time and effort, not only to make time for them in your life, but also to explain to them about your sport and your ambitions. Taking the time to do this is important.

Hobbies

Can you imagine doing nothing else all day every day but train for your sport? It might sound like fun for a couple of days, but after that it would probably get boring. It is not a good idea to concentrate on your sport to the exclusion of everything else, whatever your age or level of performance. Although there will be short periods when this might be the case, there will be plenty

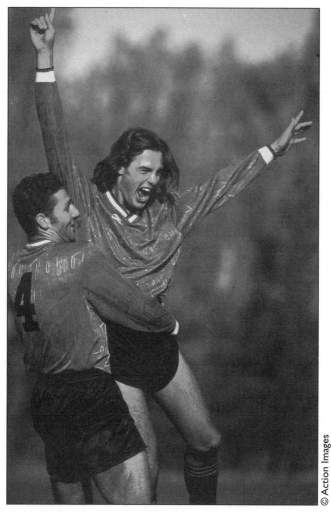

© Action Images

It's important to make time for your friends. They can help you overcome your disappointments and share in your successes.

of times when having other things to think about and do will be important; for example,

- if you become injured and have to take time off from sport,
- to help take your mind off things in the run-up to a major competition, or
- when you are taking a well-deserved rest from serious training.

Remember, a life outside sport is important. Not only will it provide you with other interests and experiences, it will help ensure that you do not become burned out by your sport before you have the chance to achieve your potential. Unfortunately, there are too many examples of elite young performers devoting their lives to sport from an early age, then, through injury or general burn-out, stopping altogether before they reach their peak because sport is no longer fun and has become too stressful. Don't let this happen to you. The next task will help you ensure that sport remains important but does not take over your life.

Task 7   Balancing Sporting, Scholastic and Social Events

Go back to Task 3 (page 9) and add important dates in the bottom three rows: school (exams, concerts), social (family occasions, friends' special events, holidays) and other (anything else that is important to you).

Check to see how they all fit together. Do the major sport competitions clash with school exams or family occasions? Does the proposed training camp clash with a possible week-end party with friends?

If there are potential problems, act now and talk to the appropriate members of *Team You:* your coach, teacher or parent or guardian.

Designing Effective Training Sessions

To help maintain a balance between your sporting life and the rest of your life, it's important to know how to make every training session as effective as possible. Success in sport is not just about training hard, although to become an elite performer there will be times when you have to train very hard physically, mentally and technically. To achieve success, whether that is becoming a world champion or simply the best you possibly can, you need to *train smart*. Learning to train smart will ensure that whatever you achieve, you will be satisfied that you fulfilled your natural potential.

Training Principles

To make your training sessions as effective as possible, you need to understand the factors that produce the best possible training effect. These include ensuring that your training is specific, at the right level and varied, and that you train regularly but take sufficient rest time to allow your body to recover and benefit from the training.

Training must be specific. The greatest improvements in fitness, mental skills or technique are achieved when training is as specific as possible to your sport and your event or position. For example, if your sport involves running, the best physical training would involve running rather than cycling, rowing or swimming. If your sport involves quick changes of direction, it is better to train in this way rather than sprint in straight lines. Training sessions that match the specific demands of your competitive sport are the most effective.

Overload your system. To improve your mental or physical fitness or technique, you need to work your body and mind slightly harder than normal. In other words, you have to overload the system to force it to adapt to a higher load. For example, if you are running, you should run at a pace that causes you to breathe harder than usual. If you are strength training, you need to work with a weight that is slightly heavier than usual. You need to work at the right level to create a positive training effect.

Train progressively. If you train at the same intensity all the time, you are unlikely to improve because your body and mind simply get used to it. As you become more physically and mentally fit, you need to make your training sessions harder. Making sessions harder as you become more fit is called *progression*.

Balance hard and easy training. It is not always possible to train hard, especially physically. When you train hard, you place your body under considerable stress and actually cause some soft tissue to break down as you overload it. Hard training sessions must therefore be followed by easier ones, because these allow your body not only to recover, but also to become more fit as it adapts to the hard training. During the easy/rest periods of training, your body recovers and adapts to the demands placed on it during your hard training sessions, allowing you to train harder next time. Hard training alone will not make you more fit. Instead, it is likely to cause a condition called *overtraining*.

Rest is vital. It is during easy and rest periods that your body actually adapts to the load previously imposed through hard training.

Vary your training. It is important to vary your training sessions. For example, if you have a choice of six different sessions to improve a particular technique, you should try a different one each time. By varying the sessions, your physical and mental fitness and your technique will improve because you keep challenging your body in slightly different ways. Also, if you keep varying the sessions, you will have more fun and training will not become boring.

Train regularly. The improvements you get as a result of training don't last forever. If you stop training, you will start to lose the fitness and skills you have gained. It is important to continue with training programmes rather than stopping and starting.

Weekly Planning

Now that you know the most important factors behind effective training sessions, it is important to incorporate them into your own programme. Understand, however, that following a training programme is not always as easy as it sounds. As you have begun to realise from the last task, you have to fit your training around all your other commitments, such as school, work, hobbies, family and friends. You may also have to find the right places to train, decide whether to train if you feel tired or decide what to do if you have to miss a training session. To deal with these problems, you need to know how to manage your training. This means knowing how to organise your weekly training and what to do or whom to ask when potential problems arise.

By knowing how and when to do your training, you will gain maximum benefit from it. This means you will improve more quickly and will reach higher levels of performance. Knowing what to do in certain situations may also prevent you from getting injured. For example, you want to avoid getting injured from doing too much fitness training or the wrong type of technical training.

When you have a lot of training to fit in, it is advisable to sit down at the start of the week and think about what you can do and when. Create a timetable and write down all your weekly commitments, such as school, sport and social activities. Then decide on which days and when you will be able to train. When doing this, remember that training does not just mean physical training; it also means mental and technical (or skills) training. Task 8 will help you plan your daily and weekly commitments.

Task 8   Planning for the Week

First fill in all your weekly commitments for school, sport (e.g., matches, fixed training times) and social activities.

Week beginning:_____

	Before school	Morning	Lunchtime	Afternoon	Evening
Mon.					
Tues.					
Wed.					
Thurs.					
Fri.					
Sat.					
Sun.					

Next identify what personal training (physical, mental, technical) you want to do and where each fits best.

Take a look at the Tips for Weekly and Daily Planning (page 26).

Now share this with your coach and seek further help on what the priorities are and exactly what training should be done.

Tips for Weekly and Daily Planning

- Always allow at least 1 day of rest from physical training each week.
- Follow hard training days with easy or rest days.
- Work on your mental skills on rest days or when your physical training is easy.
- If you are physically or mentally tired, you are unlikely to benefit fully from your technical training.
- Do not try to train hard on days when you have other commitments such as school, family or social.
- It is better to undertrain slightly than to train too much; quality is more important than quantity.

You may find that a lot of people start giving you different advice about what you should do in training. It is important to have one person who oversees and co-ordinates your training. This person should be your main coach, and you need to let this coach know who else is giving you advice and what else you are being asked to do. You may find, for example, that your physical education teacher at school wants you to take part in a competition that clashes with one for your club or simply creates another sport commitment in your busy timetable. Your weekly planner will help you identify where you have potential conflicts. Make sure you talk to members of *Team You* – your coach, parent or guardian and teacher – about any conflicts that arise.

Once you have completed your weekly planner, put it in a place where you can see it regularly (e.g., your bedroom wall or mirror). This will help you stick to your programme. However, remember that it does not matter if you miss the odd training session. Do not become obsessive about having to fit in your training because it is written on your training chart. You will not lose your skills or fitness if you miss a couple of sessions over a few weeks because of illness, tiredness or time pressures. What you have produced is a plan to guide your training; it should not be adhered to so rigidly that important things suffer or you fail to listen to your body.

Common Training Questions

The following are some frequently asked questions that relate to the training principles and the smart training advice.

Should I train near to a competition? In the 3 or 4 days before an important competition, you should reduce the amount of physical fitness training you are doing. This will ensure that you are fresh to compete and do not feel tired or heavy-legged. You should continue with your mental and technical training, concentrating on the skills you will need in the competition.

Should I train if I feel tired? If your body is tired from doing a lot of training or competing, it is not a good idea to do a hard physical or technical training session. Instead, do an easier session or take time off until you feel fresh and ready to train hard again. If you are feeling tired, you may find some mental relaxation training beneficial.

Should I train if I am injured? If you are injured, you should not do any physical or technical training that might make it worse. For example, running when you have a leg injury is not advisable. However, you may be able to do certain types of training while injured to help maintain your fitness. For example, you might be able to swim with a leg injury (for further information on this topic, see chapter 6). If you do suffer an injury and cannot train physically or technically, use the time to work on your mental skills.

Warming Up and Cooling Down

Do you always warm up thoroughly and take time to cool down properly? In addition to following the training principles described in the last section, you also need to look after your body by warming up thoroughly before training (or competitions) and cooling down afterwards.

Warm-Up

A warm-up is a set of activities you do before the start of a training session or competition to help prepare your body and mind for the exercise to follow. It is important because it

- starts to get your heart and lungs working harder, ready for when you begin to train or compete;
- warms your muscles and connective tissue (e.g., tendons, ligaments), making stretching easier and safer;
- helps reduce the risk of injury because your body has been prepared to work hard; and
- helps prepare you mentally for the forthcoming competition or training.

A good warm-up normally lasts 20 to 25 minutes (but may vary from sport to sport) and should always include three phases:

Phase 1: Continuous low-intensity exercise such as jogging or skipping that starts off gently but gets harder as the warm-up progresses. During this phase, you raise your pulse gradually so you are breathing harder and starting to feel warm or sweating lightly. This should last 5 to 10 minutes.

Phase 2: Flexibility and mobility exercises that help reduce the risk of injury, as well as prepare your muscles and associated tissues for the more extreme movements required when you start training or competing. This should also last 5 to 10 minutes.

Phase 3: Sport-specific activities (e.g., short sprints, turns, jumps and shots) that rehearse the physical and mental activities involved in the sport, preparing you both physically and mentally.

Cool-Down

A cool-down is a set of exercises you should do after a training session or competition to help your body return to its normal resting level and to accelerate recovery. Cool-down is important because it

- allows the energy systems to wind down gradually;
- helps get rid of by-products such as lactic acid that can cause muscle soreness and delay recovery;
- allows you to stretch while still warm, which is important for reducing the soreness you will sometimes feel the day after training or competing; and
- provides a great regular opportunity for you to work on improving your flexibility while the muscles are still warm.

Cool-down should last for 10 to 15 minutes. Begin by putting on some warm and dry clothing. Start with some light, rhythmical activity such as jogging or walking, gradually reducing how hard you are exercising. Follow this with some stretching exercises, particularly of the muscles used in the activity (if time permits, this is where you can extend the session to develop your flexibility).

Key Points

- Maintain a balance between your sporting life and the rest of your life with careful planning and good communication.
- Identify *Team You*—the people who help you with your sport and help keep your life balanced.
- It's important to make time for your friends, family, sport and school.
- To give yourself more time to do things other than sport, you need to train smart. This means planning each training session so that it's as effective as possible.

Improving Mind and Body

Be prepared for set-backs. What makes elite athletes is often not just how hard they train, but how well they cope with and fight back from the inevitable setbacks that occur on the way.

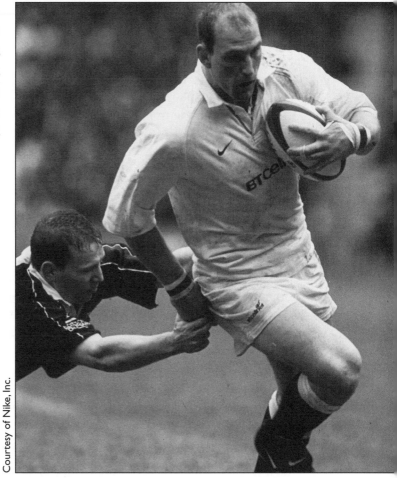

Courtesy of Nike, Inc.

Although fitness is important to most sports, there is often little difference between the fitness levels of elite athletes – on their starting blocks before an Olympic final, in a Wimbledon final or even in a national road race. What sometimes seem to make the difference between winning and coming in second are less obvious factors such as attention to detail in preparation (e.g., diet and hydration, resting to allow injuries to recover fully) or the mental toughness of the athlete to cope when things go wrong (mental skills).

In this part, you will have a chance to look more closely at four important areas that can make a significant difference in your performance: fitness, diet, mental skills and injury prevention and rehabilitation. All too often, athletes take some of these things for granted and don't work on them. They fail to believe that what they eat will make a difference in their ability to train hard and recover fully; they imagine that by competing regularly they will get fit; they assume that mental skills are inherited rather than developed like any fitness and technical skills; they think getting injured is just a matter of bad luck or that tough athletes play through an injury. These ideas don't make sense, and if you pay just a little more attention to these important areas, it will pay dividends in your performance.

Most athletes accept that they need to be physically fit to be successful in their sports. However, fitness is very specific, so it is important that you do the right sort of fitness training. The type and quality of training that you do will be more important than the quantity. Chapter 3 (Getting Fit) will help you look at each aspect of fitness and work out what you need to be doing and will suggest ways you might go about it.

In chapter 4 (Eating Right), you will have a chance to examine what you eat and compare this with what you should eat. You will probably find that making a few relatively small changes in your diet can have a significant impact on your performance.

How often do your thoughts or fears interfere with your performance? Do you sometimes feel you talked yourself out of a victory? Do you get frustrated because your performance varies so much from one competition to another? Do you find your mind wandering during a competition? All these problems relate to your ability to control and focus your mind on positive and relevant thoughts – those that make a difference to the quality of the training you do or the outcome of the competition. They can all be improved through practice, and you can get a great deal of help in doing this by working through chapter 5 (Tuning your Mind) on mental skills.

Finally, in chapter 6 (Staying Healthy), you can review your knowledge and attitude toward health and injuries – how to stay healthy, how to prevent injuries, how to cope with injuries and illness and how to recover quickly and safely from them. Time lost through avoidable injuries or illnesses can make a real difference to your sporting success. A little time, effort and thought can help you stay healthy and injury-free.

3

Getting Fit

Fitness has different meanings to different athletes, depending on the unique requirements of the sport, event or position. Many people associate fitness with sports such as marathon running. Certainly marathon running requires considerable endurance (aerobic fitness), but what about the other fitness components such as strength, power, speed and flexibility? Here the marathon runner would not do so well. You need to analyse the fitness demands of your sport and decide which have the most important effects on your performance. This will influence how you should train.

In Task 1 (page 5), you rated the importance of fitness to success in your sport. The fitness you need for performing successfully may develop partly from competing but mostly from training. Fitness is important in all sports because it can result in

- improved physical performance. If you are fit for your sport, it will have a direct positive effect on your performance.

- better recovery. Being fit helps you recover more quickly after training and competition. This might be particularly important if you need to perform again quickly, as in a tournament or an event with different heats.
- better technique. By increasing your fitness, especially your strength, you will be able to develop and maintain your skills and techniques without getting tired.
- less risk of injury. Being more fit will help lower your risk of injury, and if you are unlucky enough to get injured, the injury is likely to be less severe and you are likely to recover more quickly and fully.
- greater enjoyment. The more fit you are, the harder you will be able to train and compete without getting tired and the more likely you are to have fun.

Most sports place significant physical demands on the athlete, but these demands vary from sport to sport. Some require high levels of endurance to be able to keep working hard for a long time; others require good power for jumping and speed for sprinting; many require strength to be able to lift, throw or withstand an object; all require sound flexibility. Many sports require all these fitness components (endurance, power, speed, strength and flexibility) for success, but some may be more important than others. You need to analyse the specific physical demands of your sport, recognise the benefits of each component and learn how to train each component so you can become fit for your sport and improve your performance.

To help you in this analysis, this chapter is divided into four sections, each focusing on a specific component of fitness:

1. Developing endurance
2. Building strength and power
3. Gaining speed
4. Improving flexibility

Task 9 starts you off by helping you determine how important each fitness component is to your sport. The rest of the chapter covers ways to improve each type of fitness.

Task 9	Rating the Importance of Each Fitness Component

Go back to Task 2 (page 6) and reassess your responses to the first set of questions related to fitness. Then try to rate the importance of each fitness component for you in your sport using the following scales:

	Unimportant				Very important
Aerobic endurance	I	2	3	4	5
Anaerobic endurance	I	2	3	4	5
Strength	I	2	3	4	5
Power	I	2	3	4	5
Speed	I	2	3	4	5
Muscular endurance	I	2	3	4	5
Flexibility	I	2	3	4	5

Bear this in mind as you read through the following pages and work through the tasks.

Developing Endurance

How important is endurance for your sport? Endurance involves two components: aerobic and anaerobic endurance. Aerobic endurance (stamina, cardiorespiratory) requires oxygen, and you need it to sustain a high work rate, technical quality and concentration over the length of the training session or competition and to help you recover efficiently from competition and training sessions. Anaerobic endurance (without oxygen) is needed to produce high-intensity work bouts with limited rest intervals.

Aerobic Endurance

Do you need to be able to keep moving actively for more than 2 to 3 minutes at a time without a break? Aerobic endurance refers to your ability to maintain a moderate work rate. Aerobic means 'with oxygen'. You take in oxygen from the air you breathe, and this is used in the process of breaking down your food to provide energy. This aerobic system works well when you need to keep working at a moderate pace for some time (more than 2 to 3 minutes).

Aerobic endurance is important in most sports, because it helps you

- maintain your work rate during training and competition,
- maintain your skill level and concentration during training and competition,
- recover quickly between hard efforts when you are training or competing, and
- recover quickly after training and competing.

Aerobic endurance is required for all sports because, in addition to helping you sustain a high work rate and recover more quickly, it forms the foundation on which most types of fitness training can be developed.

How good is your aerobic endurance? You may be able to estimate this based on your ability to keep going without tiring throughout training sessions and competitions. You may also have been tested at some point, perhaps at school or by your coach. The typical tests used to measure this include the multi-stage fitness or bleep test, in which your aerobic endurance is measured by the number of stages you reach on the test; the 12-minute run, during which aerobic endurance is estimated by the distance you can run in the time; and laboratory tests (e.g., $\dot{V}O_2$ uptake tests, usually measured during a treadmill run). In each case, your individual score can be compared with your future scores.

You can improve your aerobic endurance in several ways, including steady pace runs, interval training and Fartlek sessions. Always warm up thoroughly before engaging in any of the following workouts.

Steady Pace Runs

Improve your aerobic endurance by running at a steady pace. This means a pace at which you can have a conversation with a friend or at 70 to 80 percent of maximum heart rate* if you are wearing a heart-rate monitor. Start running for 15 to 20 minutes and then build up slowly to around 30 minutes as you become more fit.

As an alternative to running, you could use any other rhythmic whole-body activity such as skipping, cycling, swimming, running in water, rowing or using a step machine. If you are training in a gym, you might want to do 5 to 10 minutes on two to three different pieces of equipment.

To improve your aerobic fitness, you need to run (cycle, row, swim, skip or take aerobic classes), working at about 70 to 80 percent of your maximum heart rate for between 20 and 30 minutes.

Interval Training

You can also improve your aerobic endurance through interval training sessions, usually on a 400-metre track or a firm grass surface. These involve

---

*Maximum heart rate can also be roughly estimated by subtracting your age from 220; thus, for a 16-year-old athlete, maximum heart rate would be estimated to be 220 − 16 = 204. Note that this is a very rough estimate, and there will be significant individual variations.

carrying out a series of hard efforts with a rest or light activity in between. An example of interval sessions might be to run hard for 400 metres, recover for 2 minutes and repeat this six times. You should be running at around 70 percent of your maximum speed, and you should aim to run each interval at the same speed. To make the session harder, you can increase the number of intervals, reduce the recovery between each or run faster – but do not try to do all three at once.

Fartlek Sessions

Fartlek is Swedish for 'speed play', and this type of training is simply an unstructured form of interval training in which bursts of hard exercise are mixed with easier ones, using a watch or by feel. For example, you could run easily for 3 to 5 minutes, run hard to a landmark (e.g., tree, lamp post, gate), walk or jog to recover, then select another landmark, and so on, for about 10 to 15 minutes before starting your cool-down. You should vary the distance you run hard; if training with a friend, you might take it in turns to select the landmarks. Alternatively, you could work hard for 2 minutes, then easy for 2 minutes and repeat this for a total of 10 minutes; then sprint as fast as possible for 10 seconds and walk for 1 minute, repeating this four to six times, followed by a short jog to cool down. Ideally you should do this on a firm grass surface, which may have some undulations or hills on it. Fartlek-type sessions can also be carried out using an exercise bike or rowing machine.

The aerobic energy system works well until you need to do more intensive work. Then it can no longer supply oxygen to the working muscles fast enough. For this, you need to use the anaerobic energy systems – ones that don't require oxygen to break down foodstuffs in the body to provide energy more quickly for more intensive exercises such as short sprints or jumps.

Anaerobic Endurance

For your sport, do you sometimes need to work really hard for a few seconds? If so, you will need to develop your anaerobic endurance (sometimes referred to as speed endurance), which provides the energy required to do repeated bouts of high-intensity work for short periods, less than 2 minutes (e.g., in short sprints or jumping). It is not easy to measure anaerobic endurance outside a laboratory, but sometimes repeated sprint tests are used and scores compared with future scores.

You can improve your anaerobic endurance through interval training and circuit training.

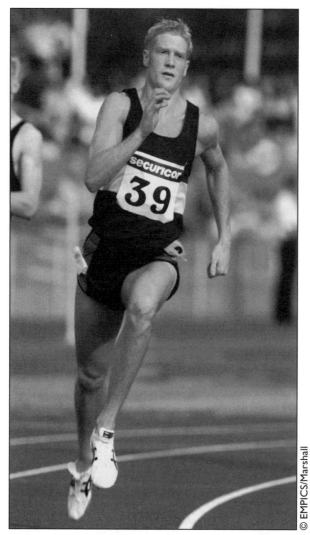

The anaerobic endurance required by athletes like sprinter Iwan Thomas can be developed through interval and circuit training.

Interval Training

Interval training can be used to develop both aerobic and anaerobic energy systems. You can help develop your anaerobic endurance using shorter, faster intervals compared with your aerobic interval sessions. You might run faster (90 percent of your maximum heart rate) for shorter distances, allowing your body to recover between each effort. For example, run hard for 100 to 200 metres, repeating this five times with 90 seconds of recovery between each run. As your fitness improves, you could increase the speed, work bouts or number of sets (the number of times you repeat the work intervals).

Circuit Training

Circuit training involves a number of stations (or activity bases), at each of which a different activity is undertaken. Athletes move from station to station in a set order and work at the prescribed activity for a set length of time or a specified number of repetitions. Circuits can be used for a variety of purposes including technical work and to develop general aerobic fitness, anaerobic speed endurance and muscular endurance. For example, you could set up 8 to 12 activity stations, working for 30 seconds with 60 seconds of rest between stations, and repeating the circuit three times. A sample circuit used by netball players is shown in figure 3.1.

As your anaerobic endurance improves, you could ensure progression by doing one or more of the following:

- Decreasing the rest period so it is equal to the work period (i.e., 30 seconds of rest)
- Increasing the work period (e.g., to 45 seconds)
- Increasing the number of sets (e.g., to four)

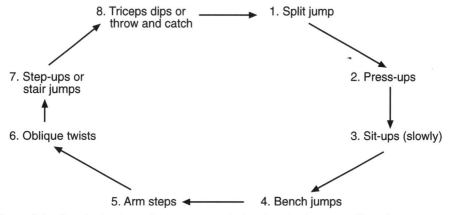

Figure 3.1   Sample circuit training programme designed to develop anaerobic endurance.

Your Endurance Needs

To help you assess your aerobic and anaerobic endurance needs, complete Task 10. This assessment will also provide you with a profile score out of 10 for each component (refer back to the self-profiling exercise you did beginning on page 11).

Task 10 Assessing Your Endurance Needs

How important is aerobic endurance for you?	Not at all	A little	Somewhat	Quite	Very
If important, how much emphasis do you place on this in your training?	None	Little	Average	Good	High
If important, how would you rate your aerobic endurance?	1 2 3 4 5 6 7 8 9 10				
How important is anaerobic speed endurance for you?	Not at all	A little	Somewhat	Quite	Very
If important, how much emphasis do you place on this in your training?	None	Little	Average	Good	High
If important, how would you rate your anaerobic speed endurance?	1 2 3 4 5 6 7 8 9 10				

Identify what you would like to improve most and how you might go about it:

Building Strength and Power

How important are strength and power in your sport? People often confuse these two terms, so it may help to start by explaining the difference. *Strength* refers to the force you can apply using your muscles. You need strength because it improves performance by making you stronger in physical contact situations and contributing to power that is important for many sports. It also helps reduce the risk of injury; if you are stronger, your muscles, ligaments and tendons will be able to take more strain before they become damaged.

Power is a combination of strength and speed but differs from strength in that it normally requires fast movements. Power is a major component of fitness in sports where you need to execute fast actions, such as in sprinting, jumping, hitting or changing direction. Improved power may benefit your performance by improving jump height and running speed; helping you to change direction more quickly; and enabling you to pass, hit or kick harder.

There is a third component to power that can also cause confusion. *Muscular endurance* is the ability to execute repeated muscle contractions without muscular fatigue. This is also a function of strength and uses the anaerobic energy systems.

Strength

For your sport, do you need to move or resist heavy objects or other performers? If so, you need to develop your maximum strength. Typically, this is measured by totaling the weight lifted once (one repetition) or, to avoid excessive strain, the maximum weight that can be lifted three times (i.e., three repetitions maximum). Some sports use a handgrip dynamometer. However it is tested, your individual score can then be compared with future scores. Strength is best developed using either resistance training (exercises in which you work against a resistance or weight) or circuit training.

Resistance Training

Resistance training is very effective but is also potentially dangerous if carried out incorrectly. For this reason, you should always work with a qualified instructor or coach to make sure you are using the right technique and that your programme is appropriate for you. Resistance training can be done using any of the following.

Body weight. Athletes should start to develop strength by doing exercises using their own or a partner's body weight as resistance. Body weight exercises include activities such as press-ups, squats and pull-ups. These exercises should be executed in a slow, controlled manner. The advantage of working with your body weight is that you can do all the exercises without equipment. It can also be a safer form of weight training, and you don't need to go to the gym.

Machine weights. Machine weights (e.g., multi-gym) are useful when you are a beginner because they help you learn the correct technique and are safer than free weights. They are usually easy to access and also tend to be quicker to use.

Free weights. Free weight exercises (i.e., ones that involve using dumbbells or barbells) work the main muscle groups but also make you work the smaller muscle groups surrounding and supporting the joint. These are called stabilising muscle groups, and they help prevent injury and improve balance. Another advantage of free weights is that you can do single-arm or single-leg exercises to help ensure your left and right sides are the same strength. This is particularly important if your sport uses one side of the body more than the other (e.g., tennis, throwing events in athletics). Safe and effective use of free weights requires very good technique that takes time to learn.

Whatever type of resistance work you do, you must train safely (don't injure yourself or someone else) and effectively (get the most out of your training sessions).

To train *safely,* you must

- always have a qualified adult with you and ensure that someone is watching or spotting for you.
- learn the proper technique and know how to do the exercise correctly (this includes getting the right breathing pattern). If you are not sure, ask a qualified instructor.
- not lift heavy weights too soon. As a young athlete, you should not lift heavy weights, as they may damage your bones or soft tissues; concentrate instead on learning good technique and co-ordination, and always follow the advice of someone experienced at developing strength in young people (an expert or your coach).
- always wear a weights belt to support your back when doing exercises that place strain on the back.
- warm up thoroughly before a session and cool down afterwards.
- never wear jewellery, always tie back long hair and always wear correct clothing (no jeans) and footwear (no day shoes).
- ensure the equipment you use is working properly and is safely secured; always check it.

Young athletes should not lift heavy weights, as they may damage bones or soft tissues; concentrate instead on learning good technique and co-ordination, and always follow the advice of an expert.

To train *effectively,* you should

- overload the muscle by working with weights that are heavier than your muscles are used to.
- always maintain the correct technique by not using weights that are too heavy.
- increase the weight slowly and progressively, once you can comfortably do 10 to 15 repetitions; then it is time for an increase.
- aim to do two to three sets of 8 to 15 repetitions for each exercise, unless your coach suggests otherwise (remember to take a rest between each set).
- work larger muscles first, working towards smaller muscles later; exercise legs, chest, shoulders, arms and then abdominals.

• start as a beginner with one session a week; as you get stronger and more used to the weights, you will need to do two to three sessions a week to improve.

Circuit Training

Circuit training can also be used to develop maximum strength. Circuit training for resistance training usually involves a series of exercises using body weight or light weights arranged in a circle. Athletes move from one exercise station to the next, performing each exercise for either a set number of repetitions or a set time. An advantage of this type of training is that it does not require a fully equipped gym, so you can make your own circuit at home.

An effective strength circuit should include 8 to 15 exercises, arranged so you do not work the same body part or muscles twice in succession. You can choose exercises that use body weight, medicine balls, dumbbells or other resistance equipment. It is important to allow enough time for each exercise or number of repetitions so the working muscles can complete the exercise but feel tired at the end of each one. Try two to three circuits with a rest period between each.

Figure 3.2 is an example of a strength circuit you could do at home.

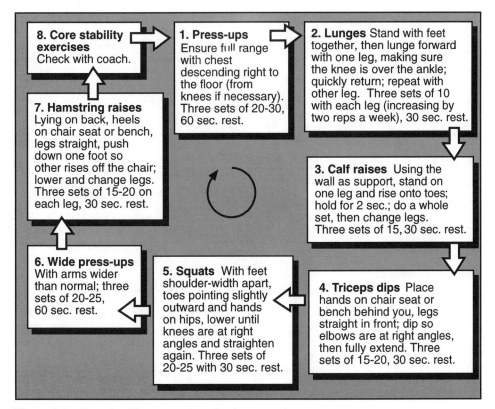

8. Core stability exercises Check with coach.

1. Press-ups Ensure full range with chest descending right to the floor (from knees if necessary). Three sets of 20-30, 60 sec. rest.

2. Lunges Stand with feet together, then lunge forward with one leg, making sure the knee is over the ankle; quickly return; repeat with other leg. Three sets of 10 with each leg (increasing by two reps a week), 30 sec. rest.

7. Hamstring raises Lying on back, heels on chair seat or bench, legs straight, push down one foot so other rises off the chair; lower and change legs. Three sets of 15-20 on each leg, 30 sec. rest.

3. Calf raises Using the wall as support, stand on one leg and rise onto toes; hold for 2 sec.; do a whole set, then change legs. Three sets of 15, 30 sec. rest.

6. Wide press-ups With arms wider than normal; three sets of 20-25, 60 sec. rest.

5. Squats With feet shoulder-width apart, toes pointing slightly outward and hands on hips, lower until knees are at right angles and straighten again. Three sets of 20-25 with 30 sec. rest.

4. Triceps dips Place hands on chair seat or bench behind you, legs straight in front; dip so elbows are at right angles, then fully extend. Three sets of 15-20, 30 sec. rest.

Figure 3.2 Example of home circuit to develop strength.

You can make the exercise harder by

- increasing the number of repetitions,
- decreasing the rest period,
- increasing the resistance used,
- increasing the number of circuits, or
- using harder exercises.

Muscular Endurance

In your sport, do you need to make repeated strong, fast movements (e.g., kicking, hitting) without a break? If so, you need to develop your muscular endurance. This is usually estimated by measuring the total number of exercises (e.g., press-ups, sit-ups, throws) performed without interruption until fatigue sets in. Your individual score would then be compared with future scores.

Muscle endurance is also best developed using circuit or weight training. By changing the exercises and the number carried out, the emphasis of the

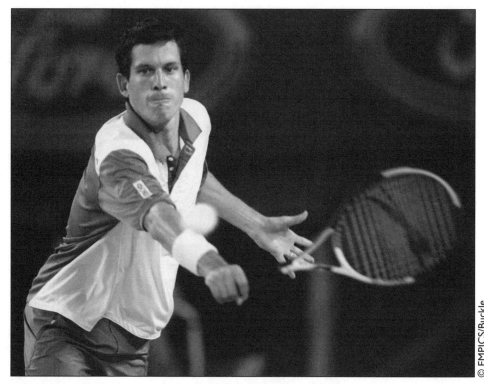

Some athletes, like tennis player Tim Henman, must have good muscular endurance to meet the demands of their sport.

circuit can be changed from maximum strength development to muscular endurance. For muscular endurance, the exercises should be executed at medium to fast speed, the number of reps should be high and the resistance low (either body weight for circuits or light weights for weight training) and two to three sets should be carried out with a rest of 1 minute or less between sets.

Figure 3.3 gives an example of a weight-training session to develop muscular endurance carried out in a multi-gym.

Name				Training aims: **Develop muscular endurance, develop lifting techniques**	
No. of sessions per week: 2				Notes: Do not lift heavy weights too soon. Always train under the supervision of a qualified instructor.	
Exercise	**Sets**	**Reps**	**Resistance**	**Speed of lifting**	**Rest**
5 min. warm-up					
Back squat or leg press	2-3	15	Moderate	Moderate-speed lift; slow, controlled return	1 min.
Leg curl	2-3	15	Moderate	Moderate-speed lift; slow, controlled return	1 min.
Dumbbell lunge	2-3	15 each leg	Body weight	Controlled descent; quick return	1 min.
Calf raise or calf press	4	20	Moderate	Moderate-speed lift; hold 2 sec.; slow, controlled return	1 min.
Chest press	2-3	15	Moderate	Moderate-speed lift; slow, controlled return	1 min.
Lat pulldown	2-3	15	Moderate	Moderate-speed lift; slow, controlled return	1 min.
Shoulder press	2-3	15	Moderate	Moderate-speed lift; slow, controlled return	1 min.
Seated row	2-3	15	Moderate	Moderate-speed lift; slow, controlled return	1 min.
Cool-down and stretch					

Figure 3.3 Sample weight-training session designed to develop muscular endurance.

Power

In your sport, do you need to make strong, fast movements such as throwing, jumping or lifting? If so, you need to develop your power. Power is a combination of strength and speed and, unlike strength, normally requires fast movements. Typically, leg power is tested by using the standing vertical jump (or sergeant jump), which measures the height jumped by the difference between your finger mark on the wall when standing and on jumping.

You can improve your power in three main ways: medicine ball training, plyometric training and weight and circuit training.

Medicine Ball Training

One way to develop power is through medicine ball training. For example, use a medicine ball (a large heavy ball similar to a 2- to 3-kilogram basketball) and execute chest passes or overhead throws to improve power in the upper body.

Plyometric Training

Plyometric training consists of jumping, hopping and bounding exercises to improve power in the legs. Plyometrics is a good power training technique involving high-impact work, but it can be dangerous and should therefore only be carried out when you have developed a really good strength base and under the strict guidance of a plyometrics expert.

Weight and Circuit Training

You can also improve your power through weight and circuit training. Weights should be lifted at speed and lowered in a slow and controlled manner. The resistance should be medium and the number of reps medium (10-15); three to five sets should be carried out with a rest of 2 to 3 minutes between sets.

Your Strength and Power Needs

To help you assess your strength, muscular endurance and power needs, complete Task 11. This assessment will also provide you with a profile score out of 10 for each component (refer back to the self-profiling exercise you did beginning on page 11).

Task 11 Assessing Your Strength and Power Needs

How important is maximum strength for you?	Not at all	A little	Somewhat	Quite	Very
If important, how much emphasis do you place on this in your training?	None	Little	Average	Good	High
If important, how would you rate your maximum strength?	1 2 3 4 5 6 7 8 9 10				
How important is muscular endurance?	Not at all	A little	Somewhat	Quite	Very
If important, how much emphasis do you place on this in your training?	None	Little	Average	Good	High
If important, how would you rate your muscular endurance?	1 2 3 4 5 6 7 8 9 10				
How important is power for you?	Not at all	A little	Somewhat	Quite	Very
If important, how much emphasis do you place on this in your training?	None	Little	Average	Good	High
If important, how would you rate your power?	1 2 3 4 5 6 7 8 9 10				

Identify what you would like to improve most and how you might go about it:

Gaining Speed

Is speed important in your sport? It is essential to many sports and can be divided into

- sprint speed, or how fast you can run (cycle, swim, row) in one direction. This acceleration speed (speed over a short distance) is crucial in sports such as netball, tennis and basketball.

- speed agility, or the ability to change direction at speed and move in many different directions. Again, this is often important in individual and team games such as squash, football and basketball.
- reaction speed, or how fast you can react or move an arm or a leg. Reaction speed is important in many games, as well as sports such as judo, fencing and boxing.

Sprint Speed

In your sport, do you need to be able to move as fast as possible in one direction? If so, you need to develop your sprint speed. This is usually measured by recording speed over a specified distance (5, 10 or 15 metres, depending on the demands of the sport). More meaningful results are obtained if you are timed using speed gates, which rely on laser technology.

Basic acceleration speed is developed through speed, power and leg strength drills; however, work should also be done on improving sprinting technique. For training to be effective, it needs to be highly specific. You should therefore be working to improve your speed over similar distances to those required when you compete. Speed is also concerned with high-quality maximal efforts, so it is important to take relatively long recovery periods between efforts (a work-to-rest ratio of at least 1:1.5). The following are examples of sprint exercises and speed running drills.

Straight-Line Sprinting

Sprint 6 x 20 metres at 100 percent effort with a full walk-back recovery. Jog easily for 3 minutes. Sprint 6 x 15 metres at 100 percent effort with a full walk-back recovery. Jog easily for 3 minutes. Sprint 6 x 10 metres at 100 percent effort, allowing a full recovery between each one.

Hill Sprints

Choose a hill that is 30 to 40 metres in length and not too steep. Run at 75 percent effort for 30 metres, concentrating on your running style, raising the knees and exaggerating the arm drive while staying relaxed. Repeat this four times with 1 minute of recovery. After a 3-minute recovery, sprint flat out for 20 metres, five times, with 1 minute of recovery.

High Knees

Skip forwards, bringing your knee high up in front; drive the opposite arm upwards; keep upright, tighten your stomach and buttocks and extend at the hips. Do this two to three times over approximately 10 metres, with a walk-back recovery after each one.

Seat Kicks

Stand tall; move forwards, taking small steps and flicking alternate heels up behind; keep the knee in line with the hip, and do not allow the hip to drift forwards; drive the arms and do not lean forwards. Do this two to three times over approximately 10 metres, with a walk-back recovery after each one.

Bounding for Distance

Run using an exaggerated action, making each stride as long as possible (bounding), with a high knee lift and arm action. Do this two to three times over approximately 10 metres, with a walk-back recovery after each one.

Speed Agility

In your sport, do you need to be able to change direction at speed? If so, you need to develop your speed agility. This refers to the ability to change direction rapidly and is important in many sports, particularly games such as netball, basketball, tennis and football. In addition to working on sprinting technique, you also need to devise agility drills based on the sort of movements you have to carry out in your sport (remember, training is specific). For example, you can set down markers and devise various movement patterns, including sprinting forwards, backwards, sideways and diagonally. Following is an example of a general drill. These drills can be timed so that improvements can be monitored over time.

Agility Exercise

Work with a group of athletes in a small area, about the size of a basketball court. One person is the tagger and must try to tag all the others. Once tagged, move out of the area. Continue until everyone is tagged. This drill can also be carried out with only one other person.

Reaction Speed

In your sport, do you need to be able to make a very quick movement in response to something? If so, you need to develop your reaction speed. Reaction speed is the ability to respond quickly and often involves rapid movement of a limb. Although your reaction speed is largely genetically determined, practice can result in some improvements. You can also learn to anticipate by identifying the relevant cues, thus appearing to reduce your reaction time. An example drill is provided below. Once again, you should devise drills that replicate the sort of rapid movements required in your sport.

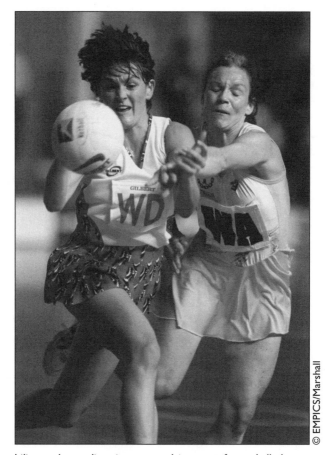

Speed agility, the ability to change direction at speed, is a must for netball players.

Reaction Speed Exercise

Your partner stands 2 metres away from you, holding a tennis ball. When you are ready, your partner drops the ball from shoulder height to one side of his body without telling you. Once the ball has been dropped, your aim is to catch the ball before it bounces. If this is too easy, drop the ball from a lower height or start farther away.

Your Need for Speed

To help you assess your need for speed, speed agility and reaction time speed, complete Task 12. This assessment will also provide you with a profile score out of 10 for each component (refer back to the self-profiling exercise you did beginning on page 11).

Task 12   Assessing Your Need for Speed

How important is straight-line speed for you?	Not at all	A little	Somewhat	Quite	Very
If important, how much emphasis do you place on this in your training?	None	Little	Average	Good	High
If important, how would you rate your straight-line speed?	1 2 3 4 5 6 7 8 9 10				
How important is speed agility?	Not at all	A little	Somewhat	Quite	Very
If important, how much emphasis do you place on this in your training?	None	Little	Average	Good	High
If important, how would you rate your speed agility?	1 2 3 4 5 6 7 8 9 10				
How important is reaction speed?	Not at all	A little	Somewhat	Quite	Very
If important, how much emphasis do you place on this in your training?	None	Little	Average	Good	High
If important, how would you rate your reaction speed?	1 2 3 4 5 6 7 8 9 10				

Identify what you would like to improve most and how you might go about it:

Improving Flexibility

In your sport, do you need to make sudden or extreme movements such as lunging or twisting, or do you need a large range of movement? If so, flexibility will be important. This refers to the range of movement at a joint and is mostly dependent on how far you can stretch the muscles, tendons and ligaments that support the joint. There are two types of flexibility:

- Static flexibility, which refers to the range of motion achieved when you move slowly (or are moved) into a stretch and then hold it (e.g., splits)

- Dynamic flexibility, which refers to the range of motion when you move quickly into a stretch using active muscular contraction and do not hold the stretch (e.g., split leap)

It is your dynamic flexibility that has the greatest impact on your performance because it determines the ease and range of movement in the skills you need for your sport. Dynamic flexibility is important for movements such as sprinting, throwing, kicking and turning; however, you should develop good static flexibility first.

Flexibility depends on factors such as bone shapes, the length of ligaments and the length of muscles. As a young child, you probably had excellent flexibility, but this may already be starting to deteriorate. Thus, it is very important that you work to maintain and improve your flexibility through stretching. Many athletes find this part of training boring and so tend to avoid or neglect doing it. However, by stretching, you can increase your flexibility, which can result in direct improvements in your performance. Flexibility is difficult to measure objectively, although certain tests are used (e.g., the sit-and-reach test that measures hamstring and lower back flexibility); however, you will notice great improvements if you work at your stretching programme.

Flexibility can be improved through stretching, and good flexibility is important for

- reducing the likelihood of tearing or straining a muscle when you move into extreme positions when performing; and
- helping you improve certain skills by allowing you to generate more power as you work through a greater range of movement and by allowing you to move your limbs more freely, which means they can move more quickly and with less effort.

Both will improve overall performance (e.g., of a tennis player's serve, a javelin thrower's action, a swimmer's stroke production).

Many athletes neglect flexibility training because they fail to recognise its benefits, which include injury prevention and direct improvements in performance.

Stretching Safely

The safest way to improve flexibility is through lengthening the muscle, and this can be done through correct stretching. You can waste time and effort if you don't know how to stretch properly, and improper stretching can also result in injuries.

Stretching should be done as part of a warm-up prior to training and competition to prepare the muscles, joints and surrounding soft tissue for the forthcoming activity. It should also be done to improve flexibility, which is the focus of this section.

Try to develop good habits about when to stretch to increase flexibility. Opportune times include those when the body is already warm (for example, after training or competition as part of an extended cool-down, during a shower or after a bath). You might also get into the habit of working on particular stretches while you are waiting for something (for example, waiting for your food to cook or standing in line for the bus).

Flexibility work takes commitment, so the following task (Task 13) may help you to make a little extra time for this important part of your training.

Task 13 Scheduling Time for Stretching

Think of occasions when you might work on a particular part of your body that needs extra time: _____

_____

_____

_____

_____

Body part: _____

_____

_____

_____

_____

Time: _____

_____

_____

_____

_____

To stretch correctly and safely, you should

- always warm up thoroughly first by performing 5 to 10 minutes of whole-body exercise such as jogging. Warm muscles stretch more easily and safely; alternatively, do stretching work under a warm shower or after a hot bath.

- lower yourself into each stretch slowly when doing static stretching exercises, and never bounce, because that can cause muscle tears.

- only stretch to a point where you feel mild tension (never pain) in the muscle.

- keep breathing normally and relax as much as possible once in the stretch position.

- hold each static stretch for 20 to 40 seconds (only 10 seconds when stretching as part of a warm-up).

- work out a stretching routine and stick to it, so you will be less likely to miss a muscle group.

- make sure you use only safe stretches (e.g., avoid stretches such as toe touching or the hurdles stretch, as these can lead to injury); if you are unsure about a stretch, check with your coach or physical education teacher.

- maintain rather than try to improve the very flexible areas (too much flexibility can increase the chance of injury); concentrate on improving weak areas.

- try to ensure that each side of your body is equally flexible, for imbalances in flexibility (or strength) can result in an increased risk of injury; work to improve the weaker side.

- always apply gentle pressure when stretching with a partner, as sudden or vigorous movements can cause injury.

Never stretch the muscles when they are cold, and always move into the stretch gently. Never bounce to increase the stretch, because that can cause muscle tears.

Static Flexibility

Following are some examples of safe static stretching exercises. You should, however, work with your coach or physiotherapist to develop other safe stretching exercises that are especially tailored for you and your sport.

Hip Flexor Stretch

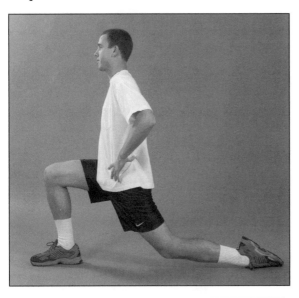

1. Take a position with your front knee bent at about 90 degrees, your other leg stretched behind with the knee off the floor and your trunk upright, hands on hips.

2. Slowly lower your back knee until it touches the floor, then gently lean your upper body backwards without arching your back.

3. Hold the stretch for at least 30 seconds and then relax.

Hamstring Stretch

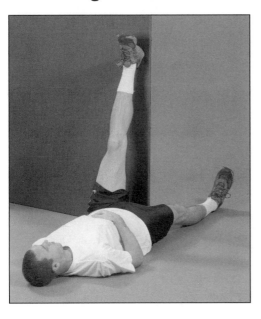

1. Lie flat on your back in a doorway.

2. Raise one leg straight so that it rests against the doorway.

3. Hold the stretch for at least 30 seconds and relax, then repeat with your other leg.

This stretch can also be done without a doorway by holding your raised leg just above the back of the knee and pulling towards your chest.

Calf Stretch

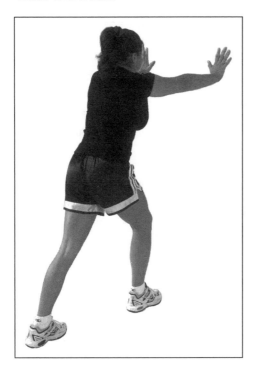

1. Stand against a wall facing forwards, your body in line, with one leg bent forwards and one straight, the foot and heel of that leg pressed into the floor.

2. Keeping this position, slide your back foot back until you feel the stretch in the middle of your calf.

3. To stretch your Achilles area, slightly bend your back leg and keep the heel in contact with the floor.

4. Hold the stretch for at least 30 seconds and then relax.

Quad Stretch

1. Lie on your side, hips slightly flexed.

2. Hold the ankle and flex that leg, bringing the heel towards your buttocks.

3. Pull the heel gently towards your buttocks while maintaining the hip position.

4. Hold the stretch for at least 30 seconds and then relax.

This exercise should be pain-free in the knee area; if you have a knee problem, avoid this exercise.

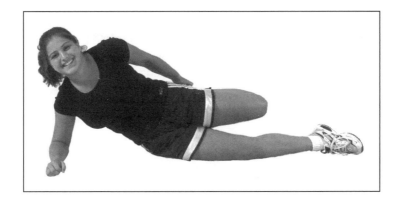

Groin Stretch

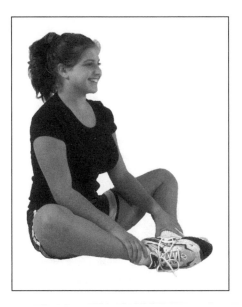

1. Sit upright on the floor with your knees flexed and the soles and heels of your feet together and pulled in towards your buttocks.
2. Place your elbows on the inside of both upper legs and gently push your knees apart with your elbows.
3. Hold the stretch for at least 10 seconds and then relax.

Lower Back and Glutes Stretch

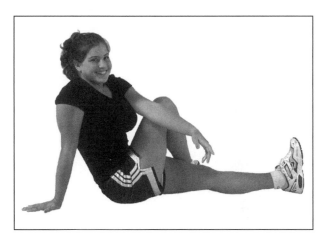

1. Sit on the floor, legs out in front, and cross one leg over the other.
2. Press the outside of the knee across your body with the back of the opposing elbow while twisting to the side of the bent knee.
3. Hold the stretch for at least 30 seconds and then relax; change legs.

Lower Back Stretch

1. Lie on your back on the floor, arms out and shoulder blades flat on the ground, one leg crossed over from the hip.
2. Press your bent knee into the floor and try to bring it close to your chest.
3. Keep your shoulders flat and your other leg straight.
4. Hold the stretch for at least 30 seconds and then relax; change legs.

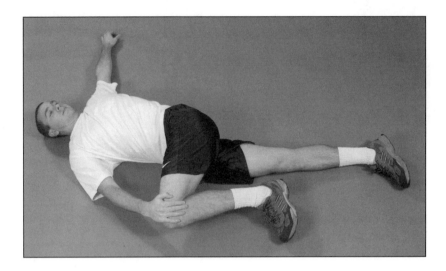

Upper Back Stretch

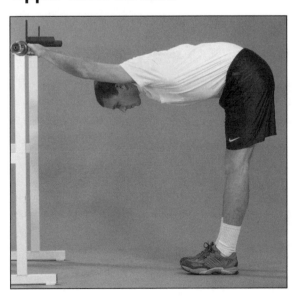

1. Using a beam or rail, stand away from it and lean forwards to grasp it with both hands, keeping your back and arms straight.
2. Keeping your waist area rigid, try to press your upper torso to the ground through your arms.
3. Hold the stretch for at least 30 seconds and then relax.

Chest Stretch

1. Stand in front of an open doorway (or in the corner of a room), one foot in front of the other, both feet facing forwards and a hand supporting your body. (Note that the two positions shown stretch slightly different regions of the chest and shoulders).

2. Slowly lean your body forwards through the doorway or into the corner.

3. Hold the stretch for at least 30 seconds and then relax.

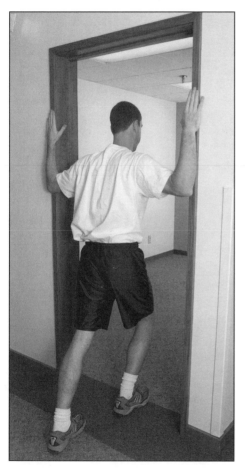 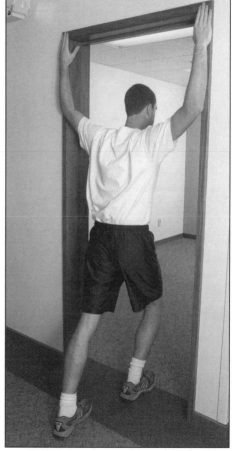

Shoulder Stretch

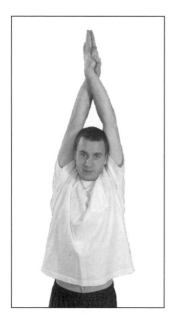

1. Stand upright, arms above your head, hands crossed and interlocked.
2. Pushing your hands together, reach upwards as high as possible, keeping your feet flat on the floor.
3. Hold the stretch for at least 30 seconds and then relax.

Triceps Stretch

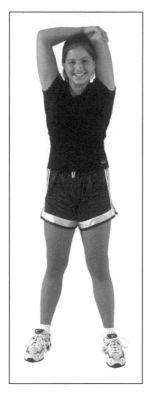

1. Stand upright with one arm flexed and raised overhead next to your ear, the hand resting on your shoulder blade.
2. Grasp your elbow with the opposite hand and pull your elbow slowly behind your head.
3. Hold the stretch for at least 30 seconds and then relax.

Dynamic Flexibility

To improve your dynamic flexibility, you must carry out dynamic as well as static stretches; however, this should be done only when you have developed good static flexibility and in conjunction with your coach.

In addition to the general stretching advice provided, when working on dynamic flexibility,

- only select dynamic stretches that are relevant to skills and movements required in your sport.
- do not use excessive swinging movements during dynamic stretches; all movements during the stretch should be controlled.
- do not bounce during dynamic stretches; all movements should be smooth and continuous.
- you should not hold the static stretch at any point; there should be continuous motion.
- ensure that you adopt the correct posture and body position during the dynamic stretches.
- if you use an implement in your sport (e.g., badminton racket), do some of your dynamic stretching with it.
- work with your coach or physiotherapist to learn this type of stretching.

Your Flexibility Needs

To help you assess your needs for improved flexibility, complete Task 14. This assessment will also provide you with a profile score out of 10 for each component (refer back to the self-profiling exercise you did beginning on page 11).

Task 14	**Assessing Your Flexibility Needs**

How important is flexibility for you?	Not at all	A little	Somewhat	Quite	Very
How often do you stretch?	Never	Rarely	Less than twice a week	More than twice a week	Daily
How well do you comply with the preceding stretching guidelines?	Not at all	A little	Somewhat	Quite	Very
How would you rate your flexibility?	1 2 3	4 5	6 7	8 9	10

Identify what you would like to improve most and how you might go about it:

Key Points

- Analyse the specific physical demands of your sport and learn how to train each fitness component to improve your performance.
- Assess which type of endurance is most important to your sport – aerobic or anaerobic – and use the exercises in this chapter to develop that endurance.
- Add weight and circuit training to your practices to improve strength and power.
- Decide the sort of speed, speed agility and reaction time speed you need and plan your training accordingly.
- Commit time to flexibility training to improve your performance and decrease the risk of injury.

CHAPTER 4

Eating Right

Do you eat and drink the right things to fuel your training and keep you healthy? By eating the right amount of the right things, you can improve your performance and speed your recovery between training sessions and after competitions. To achieve this, you must pay attention to your eating and drinking habits for 365 days of the year – not just on those days prior to competitions.

To help your body adapt positively to and recover quickly from your training sessions, you need the right nutrients and water. This chapter will help you learn what and when you should be eating and drinking.

If you are to train regularly and recover quickly, so you can remain competitive, eating should be sensible but enjoyable. The key to getting the most from your diet is to eat more carbohydrate and limit fat and to take in enough fluids. It is also important to remember that, as a young person, your body is still growing. Therefore, you need to make sure you eat enough to provide your body with the energy it needs both to grow and to train and compete.

This chapter is divided into four sections:

1. Essential nutrients for good health
2. Fueling your training
3. Eating to win
4. Managing your weight

Essential Nutrients for Good Health

Do you know which foodstuffs to eat and which to avoid? By learning more about the composition of foods, you can ensure that your diet meets your energy needs.

The nutrients essential to good health and performance include carbohydrate, fat, protein, vitamins, minerals, fibre and water.

Carbohydrate

Carbohydrate is the most important energy provider in your diet because it provides fuel for the working muscles very quickly, yet its stores within the body are relatively small. It is found in foods such as potatoes, bread, breakfast cereals, fruit, sugar, rice and pasta. The carbohydrate that you eat or drink (e.g., in fruit juice) is stored in the muscle and liver in the form of glycogen. If these glycogen stores are low, you will find training and competing harder, so eat plenty of carbohydrate.

Alcohol is also a nutrient, as it contains energy in the form of carbohydrate. This energy cannot be directly used by the muscles, however, and alcohol also constitutes a drug. Although moderate alcohol consumption is now thought to have some health benefits, it will not enhance performance. Excessive alcohol consumption will have adverse performance and health effects.

Fibre

Fibre is a non-digestible carbohydrate and is needed to improve digestion and protect against bowel and colon illnesses. Exercise also improves digestion and bowel movements, however, so additional fibre is rarely required for athletes in training.

Fat

Fat, too, is an energy provider, but it does so more slowly than carbohydrate and is therefore not the best source for athletes. It is found in foods such as butter, margarine, fried food, crisps, chocolate, fatty meat, oils, ice-cream,

cream, cheese, burgers and chips. Even the thinnest athletes have plenty of energy stored as fat, so there is no need to keep topping up fat stores. Although everyone needs some fat in the diet, most people eat too much.

Protein

Protein rarely provides a major source of energy but is needed by the body to manufacture many tissues such as muscle, haemoglobin in the blood, hormones and enzymes. Animal protein is found in foods such as meat, fish, poultry, eggs, cheese, milk and yoghurt. Vegetable protein is found in some cereals, legumes, pulses (beans, lentils and peas), nuts, tofu and soya. Rarely are athletes found to eat too little protein; most eat too much, and any excess is broken down and stored as fat. Most athletes, therefore, need to eat less protein or maintain their protein intake.

Protein supplements are unnecessary and expensive, for you can get all the protein you need from eating different protein foods each day as part of a high-carbohydrate meal. Eating large amounts of steak, fish, chicken or cheese will not help to build huge muscles; to do that, you need normal amounts of these foods, combined with a high-carbohydrate diet and the right amount and type of training.

> If you are vegetarian and do not eat many dairy products, you also need to think about the combination of protein foods you take in throughout the day. Vegetarian protein foods do not contain all the amino acids (building blocks of protein) found in animal protein foods. You need to eat a variety of vegetarian protein foods throughout the day.

Vitamins and Minerals

Vitamins are chemical compounds needed by the body for various purposes. Minerals (including electrolytes and trace elements) include chemicals such as calcium, iron, sodium, potassium, phosphorous and magnesium. These are required in minute amounts for the healthy functioning of the body. If you eat a balanced diet appropriate to the demands of your training and competitions, your vitamin and mineral intake is probably adequate. If you think it is not, it is best to make changes in the foods you choose before you spend money on a supplement. If you are considering taking a supplement, ask your coach, nutritionist or general practitioner (GP) first; you will probably find you don't need the supplement. Some athletes like to take a multivitamin and mineral supplement as a backup. This is fine, as long as it does not contain more than the recommended daily amount of each vitamin or mineral. You should avoid taking lots of different supplements containing high dosages of single vitamins and minerals, as they can have undesirable side effects.

If you are taking supplements with unfamiliar ingredients, read chapter 8 on drugs and doping control, as some products may contain prohibited substances.

Do not use supplements to make up for a poor diet.

You must ensure you have enough of two very important minerals: iron and calcium.* *Iron* is used in the body to help transport oxygen in the blood from the lungs to the working muscles. Too little iron can lead to a condition called anaemia, which can leave athletes feeling very tired and unable to train properly. Red meat is the best source of iron. Vegetarian athletes need to make sure they regularly eat foods rich in iron (e.g., fortified breakfast cereal, sultanas, dried fruit, green leafy vegetables, lentils and whole-grain foods). Iron absorption is improved by taking Vitamin C at the same time (e.g., fresh orange juice). Tea and coffee, on the other hand, hinder iron absorption.

Calcium, found in milk and other dairy products, is important for ensuring strong bones. One pint of milk (whole or skimmed) provides most of your daily requirement. You can also gain your daily requirement from one or more of the following: cheese (1 ounce), a pot of low-fat yoghurt, sardines or pilchards (2 ounces), and bread (including naan bread, scones).

Water

It is vital to drink plenty of fluids. Get into the habit of drinking before, during and after training and competing. If you become dehydrated, it will adversely affect your performance and, in extreme cases, can also damage your health. Always drink before you feel thirsty. Good drinks to choose are fruit squashes, fruit juices and plain or flavoured water. Drinking tea and coffee and too many fizzy drinks should be avoided. The best way to tell if you are drinking enough and are not dehydrated is to check the amount and colour of your urine. It should be plentiful and a pale straw colour.

Drink *at least* 2 litres of fluids each day. Always drink before, during and after training and competing; *never* wait until you are thirsty.

Isotonic drinks (e.g., sports drinks such as Lucozade Sport or Gatorade) are fluids that have the same concentration as body fluids. They are ideal fluid replacers, even better than water or pure fruit juices.

---

*Female athletes in intensive training sometimes cease to menstruate, and this can have a knock-on effect on problems such as osteoporosis. Such athletes may require supplements of calcium and/or iron, but these should be prescribed by a doctor.

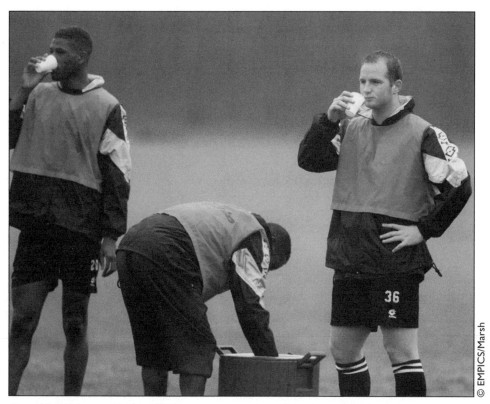

Always drink plenty of fluids to replace what you lose during training and competition.

You can make your own isotonic drinks by using

- diluted squash (one part squash to four parts water),
- diluted fruit juice (one part juice to one part water), or
- 60 grams of glucose/glucose polymer powder to 1 litre of water or diluted low-calorie squash.

Add one-fifth level teaspoon of salt to every litre of made-up drink.

Energy drinks contain more carbohydrate than isotonic drinks. Thus, they are better for replacing energy than isotonic drinks but are not as effective for replacing fluid. Some dentists are concerned that drinking too many sports and energy drinks is bad for your teeth. It is important, therefore, that you take good care of your teeth, including having regular check-ups with the dentist.

To make sure you are getting enough fluid, invest in your own drinks bottle. To stay healthy, clean it well and sterilise it regularly, and never share it with anyone. Throw away any remaining fluid after 24 hours.

Task 15 will help you assess your own diet to see if it meets your daily needs (for your sport and your body's everyday needs).

Task 15 Evaluating Your Diet

Write down everything you ate yesterday in the column below. Using the section on nutrients, try to determine the category into which each falls and place a tick in the appropriate column.

Time	Foods eaten/ fluids drunk	Nutrients				
		Carbs	Fats	Proteins	Fluids	Other

Comment briefly on what you have written down:

You should check your analysis with a teacher, sport scientist or dietician. You may want to come back and amend or add to this chart after you have read the following section on a training diet.

Fueling Your Training

Read the tips in the following chart (Task 16) and start to consider what changes you want to make to your training diet – foods you should start to eat more and foods you should eat less – by filling in the end columns.

Task 16	Making Improvements to Your Training Diet	
Tips	**Good ideas**	**My action plan**
Always eat breakfast. Breakfast is often described as the most important meal of the day; as well as providing energy for your muscles, it will help ensure that your liver can continue to supply your brain with energy throughout the day.	Cereals, toast, bread, bagels, fruit juice, boiled or scrambled eggs	
Eat within 30 min. of every training session and competition. After exercise, your muscles will be low on fuel. The best time to start refilling your energy supplies is straight after you stop, as your muscles take on energy more quickly in the first half hour.	An energy bar, energy drink, jam sandwich, scone, confectionery bar, malt loaf, bananas, raisins	

(continued)

Task 16 *(continued)*

Tips	Good ideas	My action plan
Buy your own drinks bottle. To make sure you drink enough, have your own drinks bottle and keep it topped up all the time. Do not share it, as this is a good way to pass on germs and colds (and you do not know what is in another's bottle).	If you don't have one, buy one; if it isn't named, mark it so you know it is yours.	
Keep drinking or sipping (even when you are not thirsty). As an athlete, you will lose a lot of fluids through sweating and breathing fast, so you need to drink more. It's best to drink small amounts regularly throughout the day. If you are producing plenty of clear or straw-coloured urine, you know you are drinking enough.	Good drinks to choose are plain or flavoured water, isotonic drinks, fruit squashes and fruit juices. Avoid too much tea, coffee or fizzy soft drinks.	
Eat five portions of fruit and vegetables a day. Find ones you like and think about eating some as snacks during the day. The more colourful a fruit/vegetable, the more vitamins it usually contains. Canned vegetables are good for fibre. Ask your parent or guardian to buy vegetables that are tinned in water rather than salt or sugar, where possible.	• Baked beans and sweet corn provide a lot of carbohydrate, as well as vitamins and minerals. • Bananas provide twice as much carbohydrate as apples, pears or oranges, but any type of fruit is useful. • Tomatoes, peppers, carrots and broccoli (fresh or frozen) have plenty of vitamins.	

Tips	Good ideas	My action plan
Eat enough food for your sport and body needs. As a young athlete, you will have higher energy needs than your friends who do not take sport so seriously. This is especially true when you go through a growth spurt – you have to eat enough to live, grow and do your sport. Eat snacks to help you consume enough carbohydrate.	Good snacks include: baked beans (carbohydrate and protein and hardly any fat) on toast, jacket potato, energy bars, muesli or chewy bars, banana and jam sandwiches, bread sticks, popcorn, dried fruit, jaffa cakes, currant buns and fruit scones, fig rolls, digestives, garibaldi biscuits.	
Eat foods rich in calcium and iron. Calcium and iron are the two key minerals. Calcium is needed to ensure that you have strong, healthy bones, whereas iron is a vital part of the system that carries oxygen from the lungs to the working muscles.	Milk, cheese, dairy products, lean meat, spinach, raisins, refried beans, cereals	
Eat more carbohydrate. Carbohydrate provides the best energy source for your muscles, so eat plenty (over half your calories should come from carbohydrate).	In addition to potatoes, bread, breakfast cereals, fruit, fruit juice, rice, pasta and vegetables, the following are also high in carbohydrate: rolls, bagels, pitta bread, malt loaf, scones, tea-cakes, English muffins, crumpets and Scotch pancakes, sugar, energy bars.	

(continued)

Task 16 *(continued)*

Tips	Good ideas	My action plan
Avoid high-fat foods. • Check the fat content on the food label (even foods labelled as low fat can still have a high fat content). • Ask your parent or guardian to grill rather than fry or roast.	Use sauces that are low in fat (usually the tomato-based rather than white sauces). Try to avoid croissants, doughnuts and American muffins. Try to buy the leanest red meat available, and trim off all visible fat. Take care with ready meals, including frozen fish, as these sometimes contain a lot of fat. Chicken and turkey (skin removed) or tuna (in brine or water) are good options. Low-fat crisps often have quite a high fat content despite their low-fat claims; try to eat snacks with less than 6 g. of fat per packet.	

Eating to Win

In addition to considering your training diet, which allows you to train and prepare for competition, you also should think about what you eat just before, during and after you compete. It is important to make sure you start the competition with good energy stores and are well hydrated. In some sports, you may be able to eat and drink during the competition to boost energy levels and maintain hydration. It is equally important that you consider what you eat and drink afterwards so you recover quickly and fully. During training is the time to practise any eating and drinking strategies you want to use before or during a competition. Don't try anything new on the day of the competition.

The next table (Task 17) provides some good advice about what to eat the night before, on the day of, during and after competition. This task provides a good way to evaluate your current eating habits.

Task 17 Planning Your Competition Diet

Tips	My action plan
The night before competition . . . • Eat a high-carbohydrate meal based on foods such as pasta, rice, potatoes and bread (e.g., spaghetti bolognese, chilli con carne, jacket potato with beans or tuna, pizza with salad, rice or pasta salad with lean cold meat and bread). • Drink extra fluid with and between meals. • Make sure you have high-carbohydrate snacks and drinks ready to take with you to the competition. Don't rely on suitable foods and drinks being available.	**The night before competition, I will:**
The day of competition . . . • Eat a high-carbohydrate breakfast. It is important to have some carbohydrate before you compete. Suitable breakfasts include cereal or porridge and low-fat milk, toast, bagels, crumpets, muffins with fruit juice, scrambled eggs on toast. • If you don't feel like eating because of nerves, have a drink containing carbohydrate instead (e.g., orange juice, a low-fat milkshake, an energy drink). You may find that you can manage a small snack such as raisins or currants a few at a time. • Don't leave more than 2 to 3 hr. between eating and competing. You will know from trying out new food and drink strategies during training how close to competition you can eat and feel comfortable. • Drink plenty of fluids. Try to drink up to the beginning of competition. Squash, diluted fruit juice, water and isotonic drinks are best. Avoid caffeinated beverages like tea, coffee, cola and hot chocolate. Take a drinks bottle filled with an isotonic drink to the competition.	**On the day of competition, I will:**

(continued)

Task 17 *(continued)*

Tips	My action plan
During competition . . .	**During competition, I will:**
• If it is possible to eat during the actual competition (e.g., in breaks, at half-time), bananas, dried fruit and cereal bars are good choices, as they are high in carbohydrate, low in fat and easily digested.	
• If you are able to drink, what you drink should ideally contain some carbohydrate and a little salt. As well as helping to keep you well hydrated, the carbohydrate will replace a small amount of energy, and the salt will help you absorb the fluid. Try to drink more on hot days or when competing in a hot environment.	
• If there is less than an hour between competitions, you probably won't be able to eat anything, so try to have a carbohydrate-containing drink. If there are 1 to 2 hr. between competitions, you should consider having a light snack as well as a drink. If there are more than 2 hr., have a sandwich and/or a snack and a drink.	
After competition . . .	**After competition, I will:**
• Eat a high-energy snack as soon as possible. It is very important to start your recovery straight away by replacing the fluid and carbohydrate you have used. This is when your carbohydrate (glycogen) levels will be more easily replaced as your body tries to recover.	
• You should have some carbohydrate within 30 min. of finishing a competition. Suitable snacks include bananas, dried fruit, cereal bars, low-fat biscuits, malt loaf, boiled sweets and jelly babies, as these are easily digested. If you don't feel like eating, have a drink containing some carbohydrate (e.g., fruit squash, fruit juice or an isotonic drink).	

Tips	My action plan
After competition . . . • Try to eat a main meal containing carbo-hydrate (pasta, rice or potatoes) within 2 hr. Drink small amounts and often after you have finished competing until you are producing a pale-coloured urine.	**After competition, I will:**

Managing Your Weight

The key to weight loss or gain is through a combination of dietary changes and hard training.

Weight Loss

Weight loss for an athlete who is training hard is different from a normal slimming diet because you still need to make sure you eat a lot of carbohydrate to give you the energy to do your training. What you need to do is reduce your calories by taking in less fat and protein but still taking in plenty of starchy carbohydrate foods such as potatoes, rice and pasta and avoiding sugary foods such as sweets and sugary drinks. To do this you need to

- eat fewer crisps, chocolate, pies, pasties, sausage rolls, creamy sauces/curries and fried foods;
- use low-fat spread instead of butter or margarine and low-fat milk, yoghurt, mayonnaise and cheese;
- choose lean meat and skinless chicken and turkey;
- use small amounts of oil in cooking;
- grill, bake, microwave, steam, casserole, poach or barbecue foods; and
- have mashed, boiled and jacket potatoes more often than chips and roast ones.

Do not try to maintain a fat-free diet, as small amounts of fat are essential for providing fat-soluble vitamins.

Do not try to lose more than 1 to 2 pounds a week or you will likely not be eating enough to fuel your training. Cut down, but do not eliminate, the fat and protein in your diet, and keep your carbohydrate intake high.

When athletes become obsessed with weight, the obsession starts to reduce, not improve, performance, and it can also negatively affect health and relationships. If you believe you're beginning to focus too much on your weight, ask a doctor for help before you jeopardise your health, sport performance and social life.

Weight Gain

Weight gain to increase muscle weight and bulk can be achieved by eating extra calories as carbohydrate. Together with appropriate training, this strategy results in weight gain by increasing the size of your muscles. You do not need to eat huge amounts of protein, and you do not need to take expensive protein supplements. All the protein you need can easily be provided by eating a mixture of protein foods each day, as part of a high-carbohydrate meal. If you have a poor appetite, try to eat more often during the day. You may want to have a milkshake or concentrated carbohydrate drink between meals to help provide some of the extra carbohydrate you need.

Eat more carbohydrate to fuel extra training when trying to gain weight. Aim to gain no more than 1 to 2 pounds a week, or this is likely to be fat, not muscle.

Your Dietary Needs

To help you assess your need to improve your diet or fluid intake, complete the next task. This assessment will also provide you with a profile score out of 10 for each component (refer back to the self-profiling exercise you did beginning on page 11).

Task 18 Assessing Your Dietary Needs

Question	Answer	Action
What high-carbohydrate snack do you take with you to eat after training or competition?		
How often do you use a drinks bottle and what do you put in it?		
Do you ever feel thirsty during training?		
How much do you drink in a normal training day?		
What high-carbohydrate foods do you eat regularly?		
What high-fat foods do you eat regularly?		
What one change could you make to your every-day diet that would make it a better training diet?		
How would you rate your training diet at present?	1 2 3 4 5 6 7 8 9 10	
How would you rate your competition diet at present?	1 2 3 4 5 6 7 8 9 10	
How would you rate your rehydration strategy at present?	1 2 3 4 5 6 7 8 9 10	

Personal Action Plan

Identify what you would like to improve most and how you might go about it:

Key Points

- Eat the right amount of the right foods to improve performance and help recovery between training sessions and after competitions.
- Essential nutrients for good health include carbohydrate, fat, protein, vitamins, minerals, fibre and water.
- Assess your diet to see if it is appropriate for your sport and your body's everyday needs.
- If you have a competition, think about what sort of foods to eat the night before, the day of, and during competition.
- The key to managing your weight is through a combination of dietary changes and training.

CHAPTER 5

Tuning Your Mind

Do you know how to get yourself in the right frame of mind to perform your very best? Can you reach that state when you want to? You often hear people talk about mental toughness in referring to the truly great athletes – sportspersons who seem to have the grit and determination to train hard, to win against all odds, to fight back when they are down, to stay in control when the pressure is on, to exhibit good sportsmanship and to be successful over and over again. Have they always had these positive sporting attitudes? What do they have or what have they learned to do to help them perform consistently well just when it matters most?

Although many elite athletes believe the mind is key to success, few invest as much time on tuning their mind as they do on improving their fitness and technical skills. However, with a little more thought, you could start to incorporate some mental training work, not just into your normal training, but also into other aspects of your life. The mental qualities that seem to have the greatest impact on success in sport include motivation or commitment, concentration, emotional control and self-confidence. Developing these qualities will not only help you be more successful in sport, but they will also help you in many aspects of your everyday life: in relationships, for exams, at interviews – in fact, whenever you really need to concentrate or be in control, when you have to perform at your best, when you have to deal with frustrations and disappointments or when you are upset or under pressure.

This chapter provides an excellent introduction to training your mind. It is divided into five sections:

1. Developing the right sporting attitude
2. Staying motivated
3. Setting goals
4. Improving concentration and attention
5. Controlling anxiety

Developing the Right Sporting Attitude

Developing the right sporting attitude is as important as developing your sporting ability. Taking responsibility for yourself and your actions can make the difference between success and failure. Here are some tips to help you get onto and stay on the right sporting tracks.

- Think carefully about the way you respond to others, particularly when things are not going your way.
- Think positively about all situations. Many great athletes will tell you that they learned more from their various defeats than they ever did through victory.
- Try not to blame others (e.g., parent or guardian, coach, official or team-mate) when things don't go your way. Evaluate your own performance and learn from it.
- Be supportive of other performers and team-mates, particularly when they are having a bad day. Think how you would want to be treated in the same situation.

Your Behaviour

When it comes to projecting a positive sporting attitude, your actions make all the difference.

- Thank your coach after training sessions. Most coaches are volunteers and put a great deal of their own time and effort into coaching – don't take them for granted.

- After competitions, show your appreciation to officials, even if you didn't agree with every call they made. Like you, officials may make mistakes, but they are doing the very best they can and should be recognised for their efforts.
- Take care of the equipment and facilities used in your sessions; remember, other people will need to use them after you.

Many great athletes will tell you that they learned more from their various defeats than they ever did through victory.

Coping With Success and Failure

Coping with failure is tough. It takes courage, determination and resilience to be the best. However good you are, you will encounter difficult times. The way you deal with these difficult times will determine how far you go in sport.

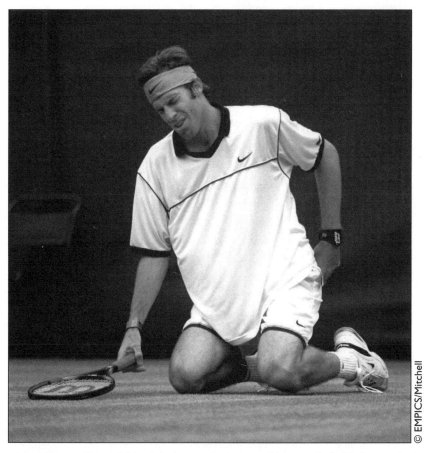

Everyone experiences disappointment during sporting careers. How you deal with these setbacks will determine how successful you'll be.

No-one likes losing, but the great athletes see it as an inevitable part of the pathway to the top. Winning gracefully can also be challenging. In the excitement and emotion of victory, it's easy to forget that your opponent is suffering. To win an important event in sport is an exhilarating, wonderful moment, and one you will probably experience. Take pride in all your achievements, but remember all those who made it possible – including your opponents.

Getting to the Top

Many athletes dream of being successful – playing at Wembley, winning a world title, winning an Olympic Gold – but what are you willing to do to get there? Many people take part in sport, train hard, perform well and achieve success. Some are tempted to cheat to reach the top. Setting your goals and dreams should not just be about what you want to achieve but also about how you intend to do it. This is something only you can decide. Discuss this with friends and consider the consequences of cheating – for your sport and for you.

> Setting your goals and dreams should not just be about what you want to achieve but also about how you intend to do it. This is something only you can decide.

Staying Motivated

Do you have to train hard to be successful in your sport? Do you sometimes find it hard to stay motivated? Motivation is one of the key mental qualities that seem to be of paramount importance to sporting success. Why is motivation so important? At a basic level, the importance of motivation is easy to understand. If you are not driven and determined to do all of those things that are going to help you become an elite performer, then there is little point in reading on. It's as simple as that. You need a great deal of motivation to succeed, but there is more to it than that. There are some important questions to answer:

- Why am I doing all this training and competing?
- What is actually motivating me to work so hard?
- What do I really want to achieve from my sport?

All these questions ask for the reasons or motives behind your participation in sport. What makes up your motivation in sport is equally important to the amount of motivation you have. It helps to understand your motives. There are two types of motives: performance motives and outcome motives.

Performance Motives

Elite performers tend to possess a high number of performance motives. This means that their motivation to compete and train is driven from inside themselves by the consistent need to develop and display their personal skills to a higher level. A high number of performance motives means that they have a high level of performance motivation.

Performance motives may include

- performing to the best of one's ability,
- mastering skills,
- enjoying the thrill of competition,
- having fun while working hard,
- challenging and improving one's skill levels,
- reaching one's full personal potential, and
- persisting and persevering through bad patches.

All these motives are personally controlled by the athlete, and no-one else has anything to do with them. Athletes with a high level of performance motivation feel a sense of achievement if they perform to the best of their current abilities and show improvement.

Outcome Motives

Many elite performers also have outcome motives that are important for them to achieve. This means their motivation to compete and train can also be driven by the need to win or overcome the opposition, sometimes regardless of how well they actually perform. If they have a high number of outcome motives, this means that they have a high level of outcome motivation.

Outcome motives may include

- achieving the status of being No. 1 in the world,
- showing higher levels of ability than the opposition,
- proving to the coach that you can win,
- gaining respect and social status from other performers by beating certain players, and
- ensuring that you win in order to please your parent or guardian.

Many elite performers are motivated by the need to show themselves and others that they are superior to the opposition. Rare is the performer who doesn't gain any sense of achievement, excitement or satisfaction from overcoming the opposition in team or individual competitions. After all, this is sport, and it is natural to be competitive. However, although it is completely natural to have outcome motives in sport, it is vitally important that performers develop and possess performance motives as well. Having outcome motivation without performance motivation does not lead to a healthy mental profile.

Performers will never win unless they can first take care of their performance. If you have outcome motives, make sure you also have performance motives. If you are not motivated to develop your performances to a higher level, then you won't win anyway.

> Outcome motivation without performance motivation leads to an unhealthy mental profile that is unlikely to result in the achievement of your full potential and long-term success in sport.

Discovering What Motivates You

Find out which type of motive (performance or outcome) is stronger in you by completing Task 19.

Task 19 Discovering Your Motives

Answer the following statements by circling how important the statement is to you on a scale of 1 (not at all important) to 5 (very important):

In my sport, to feel successful and satisfied, it is important for me to:

1. perform to the best of my current ability.	1	2	3	4	5
2. beat the opposition.	1	2	3	4	5
3. make progress in the execution of skills.	1	2	3	4	5
4. prove to others that I am better than the opposition.	1	2	3	4	5
5. give my all to perform to a high level.	1	2	3	4	5
6. show other people that I am the best.	1	2	3	4	5
7. perform stronger and better than before.	1	2	3	4	5
8. reach standards that exceed those of the opposition.	1	2	3	4	5
9. set new standards of personal performance.	1	2	3	4	5
10. perform to a higher level than my opponents.	1	2	3	4	5

Add up scores 1, 3, 5, 7 and 9 to obtain your performance motivation score.
 Performance motive:

Add up scores 2, 4, 6, 8 and 10 to obtain your outcome motivation score.
 Outcome motive:

How did you score?

Performance motivation
- If you scored 20-25, you have a strong motivation to improve.
- A score of 15-20 shows that you have moderate performance motivation, which is adequate but could be stronger.
- A score of less than 15 shows that your focus on personal performance is low, and this should be a lot higher.

Outcome motivation
- If you scored 20-25, you have high outcome motivation and a strong motivation to beat others. This is fine but could be dangerous unless your performance motivation is also high.
- A score of 15-20 on outcome motivation is moderate; beating others and being competitive matters to you, but it is not the be-all and end-all. Make sure your performance motivation is high as well.
- A score below 15 is low. You have a weaker focus on the importance of beating others. This can be fine, depending on the sport you are playing. Think about the importance of being competitive with the opposition in your sport.

If you have low scores on both outcome and performance motivation, you should talk this through with your coach.

Setting Goals

When and how do you set your goals? Do you monitor your progress against them or forget about them? Goal setting is a mental training technique that can help you develop your mental qualities. It is a particularly good technique for increasing your motivation towards achieving something important (e.g., personal best time, selection for a team, season's best distance or score). Goals are objects, targets or aims that help you focus and direct your efforts and provide the drive to help you work hard to achieve them.

Suppose you set yourself the goal of being able to run a mile in 6 minutes in 2 months' time. Setting the goal might cause the following positive changes because you

- work harder on your training, investing high levels of mental and physical effort,
- improve your concentration and pay attention to the challenge,
- develop strategies and plans about how to achieve the goal within the time, and

- solve problems in the face of difficulties because you are focused on reaching the target.

Goal setting will help you reach higher levels of personal performance. You should be able to set goals to help you improve all aspects of your performance (e.g., technical goals, physical fitness goals, mental skill goals), as well as goals in other parts of your life (e.g., schoolwork). It is important that you set your own goals; they should not be set by your coach, teacher or parent or guardian. However, all these people might help you to set effective goals – goals that are SMART. This means goals that are:

Specific. The goal you set is clear (e.g., 65 seconds for the 100-metre breaststroke) as opposed to vague (e.g., have a good race).

Measurable. You definitely know when you have achieved the goal because it tells you. For example, achieving 65 seconds is clearly measurable, but it is very difficult to measure whether you had a good race.

Achievable. It is important that the goal be challenging and difficult but still realistic for you to achieve. Don't set goals that are too difficult or too easy.

Recorded. Make sure you write down your goals in your performance diary or logbook. You can then refer back to them and feel a sense of achievement every time you look back on paper at those goals that you challenged successfully.

Time-framed. Set yourself a specific time frame in which to achieve your goals. Set long-term goals (to achieve in 1 to 2 years) and short-term goals (to achieve in 4 weeks to 4 months). Make sure, however, that you adjust the time scales if you get injured or unforeseen factors put you off course.

You can set three types of goals, each of which has its own particular purpose. These include outcome goals, performance goals and process goals.

Outcome Goals

Outcome goals are goals you cannot totally control, as they are affected by the performance of others. Typically, they are concerned with the outcome or results and include goals such as to

- win the gold medal in the 400-metre hurdles at the next Olympics,
- gain selection for the U-17 GB squad, or
- improve your ranking to 10 in the country.

However, although they are not totally under your control, they are important goals to set, particularly for the long term, because they are highly motivating.

Performance Goals

Performance goals are goals over which you have total control and responsibility, for they are not affected by other performers. Performance goals are usually personal standards of performance that you set yourself (e.g., a certain time, distance, percentage) and include goals such as to

- achieve a 46-second lap time for the 400-metre hurdles,
- pass with over 75 percent accuracy in the game, or
- make 70 percent on average of first serves in this month's matches.

Performance goals are vital stepping stones to help you achieve your outcome goals.

Process Goals

Process goals are goals that relate to the processes you need to control if you are going to achieve your performance and outcome goals. You have full control over these goals and can accept full responsibility for them. They include goals such as to

- maintain a good stride pattern between hurdles,
- release the ball cleanly to your team-mate, or
- go through your pre-serve routine before every point throughout the match.

You need to be able to set and use all three types of goals effectively. It is pointless and unhealthful to set an outcome goal without considering the pathway to achieving the goal – the pathway provided by performance and process goals. They are the foundation, and they are vital to your success. Process goals are important, for they help you achieve your performance and outcome goals by helping you focus on the way you need to perform rather than the desired outcome.

You can set goals for every aspect of performance (technical, fitness, mental). You can set goals for training and competition and make them long term (1 to 2 years) or short term (a few days, weeks or months).

Try out your skill in setting goals by completing Task 20. Ask your coach, teacher or parent or guardian to read this section on goal setting and then check how well you were able to put this important skill into practice.

Task 20 Setting Goals

Think of an event or competition that is coming up in 6 months' time and then complete the following:

What will be your outcome goal for this event?	
List three performance goals (technical, tactical, physical and mental) you need to achieve in the 6-month time to have a good chance of achieving your outcome goal:	
List three process goals you need to achieve over the next few months in training and competition that will help you achieve your performance goals and outcome goal:	
How well do you currently use goal setting in your sport?	1 2 3 4 5 6 7 8 9 10

Improving Concentration and Attention

In your sport, do you need to concentrate for long periods or to concentrate, then switch off, then concentrate again? Inevitably, some form of concentration is likely to be important to you, but it isn't just about focusing better or concentrating harder.

If you imagined tennis players watching the match on the next court rather than focusing on their own match, you might say their levels of concentration were poor. Actually their levels of concentration might be very good, as they are quite skilled at focusing on the next court. The problem lies in the quality of their attention – they are attending to something that is completely irrelevant to their performances. They should obviously be attending to their own court, not the action going on nearby.

Focusing on What's Important

It helps to understand the difference between concentration and attention. Depending on your sport, it may be critical for you to be able to focus your attention for long periods and to keep refocusing your attention. However, what is even more important is the quality of your attention. How good is your mind at focusing on what matters to your performance and ignoring what is completely irrelevant and negative to your performance? Understanding attention is not easy. One of the best ways to understand attention is to consider how your mind can focus on different thoughts, feelings or objects and switch amongst all of them. Task 21 will help you to understand this.

Task 21 | Switching Your Focus

Try the following exercise:

1. Pick up a ball and focus all your attention on the writing or logo.
2. Now stand on one leg and feel the weight of your whole body balancing on one foot.
3. Now focus back on the writing on the ball, blocking out the feeling of the leg.
4. Now think of a positive statement you might make to yourself in competition.
5. Imagine yourself saying the positive statement to yourself in that situation.
6. Now focus back on the leg.
7. Change legs and focus on the other leg.
8. Now think of the strategy or game plan that you employed in your last match or competition.
9. Replay the strategy, being successful in that competition.
10. Now focus back on the ball.

In this exercise, you switched between thoughts, feelings, objects and images a number of times. Your attention switched channels, just as it does in training and competition. The key is obviously to make sure that you switch to the right channels at the right times. This can be achieved by remembering the TV guide to concentration.

The TV Guide to Concentration

As a performer, it is critical for you to focus your attention on those thoughts, feelings, objects and images that are relevant to performance. At any point in time, however, your attention can be tuned in to one of four TV sport channels.

BBC1. When you are tuned in to BBC1, your attention is focused on one or two people or objects in the environment (e.g., an opponent, the ball, a team-mate, the lane). BBC1 is an important channel during performance because you can narrow your attention to something or someone that may help you achieve your goal. In tennis or squash, for example, a player focusing on the ball or her opponent would be using the BBC1 concentration channel. Clearly, it is important to tune in to the right objects. You are using BBC1 right now by focusing on the words on this page.

BBC2. When you are tuned in to BBC2, your attention is focused more broadly on a number of factors or people in the environment (e.g., the crowd, weather conditions, other competitors, the opposing team, two or three team-mates). BBC2 is an important channel for assessing who or what is around you. However, you need to be sure to focus on what is relevant and not distracting to your performance. For example, there might be as many players who focus on the crowd to draw inspiration as there are players who become anxious and perform poorly because they worry about who is watching in the crowd. Always carefully consider whether the content of your BBC2 channel is useful or disruptive.

ITV. When you tune in to ITV, your attention has switched to one of the most important channels. ITV is about the internal thoughts and feelings you experience in competition and training. A performer using the ITV channel can employ positive thoughts, imagine successful outcomes and manage mistakes effectively. However, performers can also use this channel to focus on negative thoughts and feelings (e.g., What if I don't win? I hate playing in this position. I bet I miss this.) You need to practise getting rid of negative thoughts and replacing them with positive thoughts about the situation. Only then can you use the ITV channel in a positive manner.

Channel 4. When you tune in to Channel 4, you are switching to the strategy and game plan channel. Your attention is focused on the strengths and weaknesses of the opposition, as well as on your own strengths and weaknesses. You can use this information to develop a plan of attack, a strategy for your performance or a particular tactical move. You will use Channel 4 most frequently prior to competition or perhaps during breaks in play, when you have time to focus on your options. It is important to tune in to this channel because it will help you make the right decisions at the right times.

BBC1 – a narrow focus of attention; needs to be on the relevant external cues (e.g., the ball), not the outcome of the competition.

BBC2 – a broad focus of attention; needs to be on relevant external information (e.g., your team-mates, not the crowd).

ITV – internal thoughts and feelings; needs to be positive (imagining successful performance), not negative (What if I lose?).

Channel 4 – focusing on your strategy and game plan; using this channel effectively means you can assess what's going on, consider your options and make the best decisions.

Try doing Task 22 to see what these channels mean when you are performing in your sport.

Task 22	Tuning In to the Right Channels

Try the following exercise:	
BBC1: List the most important things on which you need to narrow your focus (e.g., objects, people, parts of your body) to be an effective performer.	
BBC2: List all the factors (e.g., objects, people, weather, score) of which you sometimes need to be aware to help your performance.	
ITV: List the positive thoughts, statements and images you can use in training and competition to help maintain self-confidence and stay in control.	
Channel 4: List your strengths and weaknesses and consider different styles of play or strategies you might use in forthcoming training sessions or competitions.	

Now that you have the contents of your TV channels, your task is to become aware of when you are tuned in to the wrong channels at the wrong time or with the wrong content. Only then can you begin to switch to the right channels at the right time with the right content.

Your Concentration Skills

To help you assess your attention and concentration skills, complete Task 23. This assessment will also provide you with a profile score out of 10 for attention and concentration (refer back to the self-profiling exercise you did beginning on page 11).

Task 23	Assessing Your Attention and Concentration Skills

How well do you keep your attention on the relevant external information and avoid any distractions (i.e., to control BBC1 and 2)?	Not at all		A little		Somewhat		Quite		Very	
How well are you able to keep your mind focused on positive internal thoughts and feelings (i.e., to control ITV)?	Not at all		A little		Somewhat		Quite		Very	
How well do you use your strategy and tactics in the competition (Channel 4)?	Not at all		A little		Somewhat		Quite		Very	
How would you rate your ability to control your attention and concentration in training?	1	2	3	4	5	6	7	8	9	10
How would you rate your ability to control your attention and concentration in competition?	1	2	3	4	5	6	7	8	9	10

Identify what you would like to improve most and how you might go about it:

Controlling Anxiety

Do you sometimes get very anxious when competing? Do you sometimes have difficulty psyching yourself up? Do you ever lose your confidence in your ability? Inevitably, most athletes feel a certain level of nervousness or worry in certain situations, and some lose confidence in their ability from time to time. When you enter competition, it is similar to entering a battle, and your mind wants to make sure you are sufficiently prepared, physically and mentally, to give it your best shot. Although some anxiety can benefit performance by sharpening attention and activating the body physically, too much anxiety can interfere with performance (e.g., loss of fluency or control). Therefore, you need to be able to control your anxiety.

There are two different types of anxiety: cognitive and somatic.

Cognitive Anxiety

Cognitive anxiety is felt when you worry about the outcome (before or during the event) and have fairly low expectations, self-doubts and negative thoughts about your performance. Your attention and concentration begin to suffer as you lose your ITV channel focus on positive thoughts. You become confused and begin to make poor decisions; your performance deteriorates quickly. The solution is to make sure you practise filling your mind with positive thoughts and positive responses to situations so negative thoughts are not allowed to enter. If you pay attention to positive thoughts, you are beginning to control your cognitive anxiety. You need to practise talking to yourself positively and making positive remarks and comments if you are to develop the ability to respond and counter any negative thought that comes into your head.

Focusing on the positives will help you overcome your cognitive anxiety.

Somatic Anxiety

Somatic anxiety is experienced when you become nervous and tense. You feel your heart beating faster, you start going red and getting flushed and you might have a sensation of butterflies in your stomach. These are all signs that you are physiologically aroused; the mind has prepared the body for action and has turned all its systems on ready for the battle of competition. Some performers want to feel the nerves, the elevated heart rate and the nervous energy; others want to feel more relaxed and calm. Performance in some sports (e.g., rugby) might be enhanced by having a higher level of physical readiness, whereas other, more technically complex skills (e.g., golf) seem to require a more relaxed physical state.

Each type of anxiety can trigger the other; if you are experiencing negative thoughts (cognitive anxiety), you are more likely to experience somatic anxiety. If the mind doubts the body's capability, the mind increases the body's arousal and energy so it can sort itself out. If you interpret an elevated heart rate as a sign of (somatic) anxiety, you will probably start to worry (cognitive anxiety) about the forthcoming performance.

The problem is that too much muscle tension and nervousness can cause all your fluency and rhythm to disappear; your performance becomes

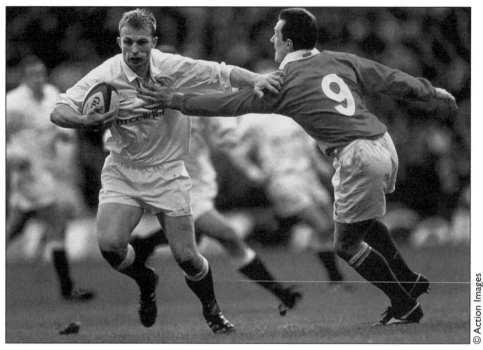

Some sports, like rugby, require a high level of physical readiness, while others require a more relaxed state.

cautious and defensive, you fail to execute movements correctly because you are stiff with tension and your legs become heavy and fatigued. Your performance becomes unnatural and uncoordinated. Thus, being able to control your somatic anxiety is a crucial skill.

Ideal Performance State

You need to become aware of your ideal performance state for your sport. What do you think and how do you feel when you are performing at your highest level? What thoughts do you have? Is your body calm and relaxed, or is it energised and psyched up? How is your self-belief or confidence? Although you need to block out negative thoughts, you also need to control your level of activation. If you can imagine the brim of a mug or cup, you need to find a state of mind and body that is full to the brim. You'll underperform if your cup is only half full and not activated enough; your performance will be poor if your anxiety floods over the brim. Getting your performance state to be at the brim involves four techniques for you to learn and try, and you can remember these through the acronym BRIM.*

---

*Developed and written by Dr. Chris Harwood, Loughborough University, Leicestershire, United Kingdom.

- **B**reathing
- **R**elaxed muscular state
- **I**magery (this is a technique used to re-create an image; for example, you might imagine yourself serving effortlessly, running the final bend, jumping to rebound the ball successfully)
- **M**atch talk

Each technique can be used either to control excessive cognitive and somatic anxiety or to increase your arousal levels if you don't feel ready for competition. Initially, they should be tried at home whenever you have some spare time, but gradually you should use them to activate your ideal state in training, then before competition and finally during the competition. By this stage, you will need to have adapted to the exercise so you can achieve the state more quickly, in about 30 seconds. However, you can learn to do this only through a lot of practice, gradually shortening the time perhaps a minute at a time, without losing the impact. Task 24 shows you how to use the BRIM techniques either to reduce or increase your arousal levels.

Task 24 Achieving a Relaxed State

Try the following exercise at home. It will probably take 15 to 20 minutes, so find a quiet place where you won't be disturbed. Because it is carried out with your eyes closed, you will either have to memorise the steps, put them onto an audiotape or ask a friend to read them to you as you respond.

1. Close your eyes and focus all your attention on the act of breathing.
2. Inhale deeply and steadily, feeling your chest rise and your rib cage expand.
3. Exhale slowly and fully, repeating the words *calm, smooth, control* or *relax* to yourself on each exhalation.
4. Feel your chest fall like a balloon deflating.
5. Continue with the process and imagine how the oxygen going to your muscles is going to help them relax.
6. Work through each muscle group (e.g., legs, arms, shoulders, feet, hands) by first tensing the muscle group and then feeling a sensation of relaxation in the muscle.
7. Try to imagine how each muscle looks when it is tense and how it looks when it is completely relaxed.
8. Continue using any positive words that help you focus your attention on the task at hand.
9. When you have finished relaxing each muscle, spend 2 more minutes focusing on your breathing.
10. Imagine yourself performing in this ideal state in competition.
11. Open your eyes when you are ready.

The BRIM exercise you have just completed will help you to reduce arousal. It should allow you to

- feel very relaxed (keep the anxiety from flowing over the brim),
- be more aware of your breathing,
- be in control of your muscle tension and relaxation,
- make use of self-talk (saying positive things to negate the cognitive anxiety and increase your self-confidence), and
- use imagery.

Once you can successfully achieve the relaxed state, start to use the techniques in training and competition situations. Of course, you will need to shorten the exercise so you can relax effectively in just 5 minutes, then 1 minute and then the recommended 30 seconds. Reduce the time gradually, ensuring plenty of practice at each time span; don't jump suddenly from 20 minutes to 30 seconds.

The next exercise (Task 25) uses the BRIM techniques to increase arousal and make you more physically and mentally activated for competition. You should use it only if you feel you need to become more physically aroused and energised for competition.

Task 25 | Achieving an Energised State

Try the following exercise during a training warm-up:

1. Focus your attention on your breathing.
2. Inhale quickly with short, sharp, shallow breaths.
3. Feel the sensation of energy, vigour and aggression with each quick exhalation.
4. Intersperse this breathing ritual with bouts of physical effort (e.g., shuttle running) to maintain a high heart rate.
5. Consider repeating emotional, confident and positive statements to yourself (e.g., I can do it, get up for it, be strong, be ready).
6. Work on releasing all the tension in the key muscles so they are relaxed and ready for action. Remember you can have relaxed muscles at the same time as being energised for action.
7. Imagine yourself in this energised, aroused, yet muscularly relaxed state during performance. Feel the sensation of strength, power, confidence and presence that you exhibit as an athlete who is totally physically and mentally prepared.
8. Continue using a combination of positive words and statements alongside imagery of a confident start in your forthcoming performance.

Using the BRIM technique may seem a little strange at first, but the principles are sound. You want to be in a situation where you are responsible for creating the mental and physical state you want to be in. You want to avoid situations where the competition makes you feel anxious and you are left to try to cope with it. It is much better to be proactive and learn how to create the ideal state than to be reactive and have to respond when you are suddenly faced with high levels of anxiety. You can also use the BRIM technique to activate your arousal levels and thus bring your activation level to the brim. The technique is summarised in table 5.1.

Table 5.1 Reaching Your Ideal Performance State		
	To relax (I'm too anxious; over the BRIM)	**To activate (I'm not up for it enough; below the BRIM)**
Breathing	Slow, deep rhythm	Fast, shallow
Relaxed muscular state	Tense and release muscles to develop the ability to relax muscles whenever required	Tense and release muscles to develop the ability to relax muscles whenever required
Imagery	Calm pictures, imagining being in control, with presence and power	Energising pictures, imagining physical control
Match talk	Relaxing cue words (calm, relax, smooth)	Powerful, emotive talk (get up for it, tough)

Task 26 helps you rate how well you are able to control your anxiety. Use the techniques in this chapter to help improve the areas in which you are the weakest.

Task 26 Assessing Your Ability to Control Anxiety

Rate your current ability to control your anxiety and build your self-confidence on a scale of 1 (very poor) to 10 (could not be better):

Your ability to control cognitive anxiety	1	2	3	4	5	6	7	8	9	10
Your ability to control somatic anxiety	1	2	3	4	5	6	7	8	9	10
Your ability to use self-talk	1	2	3	4	5	6	7	8	9	10
Your ability to use imagery	1	2	3	4	5	6	7	8	9	10
Your ability to use relaxation techniques	1	2	3	4	5	6	7	8	9	10
Your ability to control your breathing	1	2	3	4	5	6	7	8	9	10

Identify what you would like to improve most and how you might go about it:

Key Points

- Developing the right sporting attitude can be the difference between success and failure.
- Motivation is an important mental quality that will lead to success in your sport. Find out what motivates you and ways you can sustain that motivation.
- Setting goals will help you reach higher levels of personal performance. Goals give you the focus and drive to work hard to achieve more.
- As a competitor, it is important to focus your attention on those thoughts, feelings, objects and images that are relevant to performance.
- Use breathing, relaxation, imagery, and match talk to help reduce or increase your arousal levels in order to reach your ideal performance state.

CHAPTER 6

Staying Healthy

How well do you take care of yourself? How often are you injured or unwell? *Prevention is better than cure*. Have you had an injury that has kept you from training and competing? Do people encourage you to practise drills, exercises or new techniques that prevent injury? Unfortunately, these exercises and drills are often seen as boring and it's easy to ignore them and just do what you want to do. Most athletes realise they should have paid more attention to injury prevention only when they sustain an injury – and by that time it's too late. If you can remain injury-free, you can train and compete as hard and as often as you like.

To stay active and injury-free, you need to know how to keep yourself healthy, what is likely to cause injuries, what actions you can take to reduce the likelihood of injuries and what to do when injuries inevitably occur. Along those lines, this chapter is divided into four sections:

1. Looking after your health
2. Understanding the main causes of injury
3. Preventing injuries
4. Treating injuries

Looking After Your Health

Do you look after your health properly? If you look after your general health, you can reduce the likelihood of injuries and illness. In addition to ensuring that you eat sufficient carbohydrate to meet your needs (to live, grow and practise your sport), you should also ensure that you give your body enough time to recover from training. For training to have the desired effect, you have to overload the body. Too great a physical training load can cause pain, injury and ultimately overtraining or burn-out; too little will mean no gain. Remember, too, that the positive training effect comes after the physical training, while the body is recovering. It is therefore vital that you give your body sufficient time to recuperate from hard physical training. This means

- always cooling down thoroughly (few athletes devote enough time to this aspect of training);
- maintaining hydration levels and replenishing carbohydrate stores as soon after training or competition as possible;
- following very hard training sessions with easier ones;
- taking at least 1 day off a week from training and competition;
- taking advantage of recovery techniques such as alternating hot and cold showers or spa-baths, sports massages and swimming* (although these techniques should not be used as a substitute for an effective cool-down); and
- getting 8 to 10 hours of sleep a night and trying to adopt regular sleeping patterns (going to bed and getting up at the same time each day).

It is important to listen to and monitor your body so you know how it is responding to your training habits. One good indicator of fitness is your resting heart rate. You should record your resting heart rate each morning (i.e., record your pulse on waking and before getting out of bed). This provides a good indicator of your reaction to training. Decreases indicate you are becoming more fit; increases are a warning sign than your body is not

---

*Swimming is an excellent example of active recovery that can be used after training or competitions; activities might include walking in the water, backstroke and sidestroke swimming, as well as low-intensity kicking using a board.

coping with the training load. You should also record your body weight each morning (before eating and after going to the toilet); small fluctuations are of no concern, but unexplained weight loss may indicate overtraining or dehydration. Just as important is to record your attitude towards training. It is normal to feel tired after training, but continuous feelings of fatigue for several days may indicate that you are not adapting to the training load or recovering fully. If these sorts of symptoms occur, tell your coach, teacher or parent or guardian straight away.

Signs of overtraining include poor sleep patterns, increased resting heart rate, unexplained weight loss, continuous feelings of fatigue and changes to or cessation of menstruation in females.

An important part of looking after your general health means having regular medical check-ups. Dental and eye examinations are just as important as medical ones. The eyes, for example, reveal a lot about your health as well as your vision. Good vision is essential to most sports, so it is important to protect your eyes. You should

- have your eyes examined by an optometrist at least every 2 years,
- always wear spectacles if you need them (they will not make your eyesight worse),
- take regular breaks if you use a computer and ensure that the screen is just below eye level, and
- always wear a brimmed hat and sunglasses in strong sunlight.

Understanding the Main Causes of Injury

Do you know the main reasons why injuries occur in your sport? There are two main causes of injury:

- **Direct causes.** Injuries commonly occur as a result of a fall or a blow. Such injuries may be more likely to occur in high-risk activities (e.g., skiing), in poor conditions (e.g., wind, rain, slippery or uneven surfaces) or in contact sports such as rugby and those involving people or objects moving at speed in confined areas (e.g., squash, netball).
- **Indirect causes.** Tissues can be injured as a result of overuse, poor technique, unsuitable equipment, inappropriate training programmes and overtraining or under-recovery.

Although anyone can sustain injuries, some athletes seem to be more at risk than others. This may be caused by one or more of the reasons in the following chart (Task 27).

Task 27 Identifying Potential Injury Risks

Read through the following reasons and examples and then try to identify potential injury risks for you.

Common causes of injury	Potential injury risks in your sport
The specific demands of your sport: • If yours is a contact sport, you are more likely to sustain impact injuries such as bruises, fractures and dislocations. • If your sport involves a lot of repetition, such as distance running or rowing, you are more likely to sustain overuse injuries. • If your sport involves fast-moving objects (e.g., squash), consider wearing eye protection.	**Typical injuries:**
The types of training methods or practice: • Lifting weights that are too heavy or working on power before you have developed a good strength base • Fatigue: failing to allow the body sufficient time to recover following hard training sessions • Engaging in intense activity without warming up	**Injuries you have sustained (or could) for this reason:**
The developmental stage of the body (e.g., still developing): Excessive force or loads being placed on bones, muscles and tendons, especially during growth spurts	**Injuries or illnesses that have occurred (or could) for this reason:**

Common causes of injury	Potential injury risks in your sport
Undetected physical imbalances or fitness limitations: • Flexibility or mobility limitations • Lack of endurance, strength and/or power • Poor co-ordination or balance • Strengthening the powerful shoulder muscles without strengthening the muscles that stabilise the shoulder joint can make the joint more vulnerable to injury • Overuse of one side of the body (e.g., racket players) and the resulting imbalance	**Injuries you have sustained (or could) for this reason:**
Poor technique or failure to comply with the rules: Certain drills may place too much compensatory strain on other parts of your body (e.g., a breaststroke swimmer with too wide a leg kick may suffer knee injuries or a football player who dives in for the ball from behind is more likely to misjudge the tackle and cause an injury).	**Injuries you have sustained (or could) for this reason:**

Preventing Injuries

Do you take action to reduce the likelihood of getting injured? Once you are aware of the sort of factors that increase the likelihood of injuries, it is easy to identify things you should and should not do.

To prevent muscle and other soft tissue imbalances,

- ask your coach or chartered physiotherapist to assess you to identify any muscle and other soft tissue imbalances and make recommendations about specific exercises to rectify any problem before injuries occur.

- maintain good posture at all times.

- work on both sides of the body and opposing groups of muscles (e.g., hamstrings and quads, biceps and triceps).

Be patient; it may take up to 3 months to see any improvement.

To prevent injuries caused by poor technique or equipment,

- ask your coach to check your skills and training drills. Are they appropriate for your event, age, body type and stage of development?
- commit to working on a technique that is faulty, even though there may be an inevitable loss of form for a while.
- always wear the recommended protective clothing (e.g., mouth guards, shin pads, helmets) and footwear, even in training.
- look after your sports equipment and footwear. Always replace equipment, particularly footwear, when it is becoming worn.

To prevent recurring injuries, always

- ensure that you gain approval of the chartered physiotherapist or doctor before resuming training after injury.

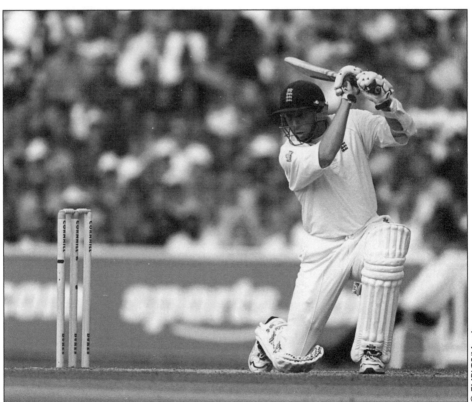

Always wear the recommended protective clothing during practice and competition.

- build up to full training gradually, and do not compete until you have regained full movement.

To prevent overuse injuries,

- always follow all the advice mentioned in the sections above.
- never exceed the training load set by your coach.
- be aware of niggling pain that may herald the start of an overuse injury and seek medical advice.

Treating Injuries

Do you take the right course of action when you get injured? Unfortunately, however well you follow the preceding advice, the chances are you will sustain an injury from time to time. Therefore, it is important to know what to do and what not to do to hasten recovery. Although injury can involve damage to several structures within the body and may be severe enough to demand admittance to a hospital, most sport injuries involve damage to the soft tissues.

Soft Tissue Injuries

Soft tissue injuries are usually categorised as

- first-degree injuries: mild injuries, where swelling, bruising and pain are slight and self-treatment is possible.
- second-degree injuries: characterised by moderate swelling and bruising, with pain on any movement; you should seek advice from a doctor or chartered physiotherapist.
- third-degree injuries: where there is a complete tear of the injured tissue, significant swelling and bruising with severe pain, even at rest; you should seek professional advice as soon as possible.

If in doubt, *always* seek advice from qualified professionals, especially for a second- or third-degree injury.

PRICE Guide

For first- and second-degree injuries (or as a first-aid measure before you seek professional advice), use the PRICE guide* for the first 3 days (72 hours).

---

* Based on *Guidelines for the Application of "PRICE" During the First 72 Hours Following Soft Tissue Injury*, which has been produced by the Association of Chartered Physiotherapists in Sports Medicine (ACPSM).

This process helps reduce the inflammation that accompanies soft tissue (muscle, ligament and joint) injuries and so accelerates the healing process. You will be able to recognise the signs and symptoms of inflammation: heat, redness, swelling, pain and inability to use the injured part normally. If the injury is not settling after 3 days, seek professional advice.

P: Protection
R: Rest
I: Ice
C: Compression
E: Elevation

Protection

Protection avoids further stress to the injury and can include

- avoiding full weight bearing (e.g., using crutches),
- general support (e.g., slings), and
- specific support for the injured tissues (e.g., braces, splints).

The protection should not be too tight, because there will probably be some swelling.

Rest

Rest prevents further damage and bleeding. Depending on the severity, the rest period may have to continue for more than 3 days. It may be possible to exercise gently the uninjured parts of your body; however, you must avoid any strenuous activity, even to uninjured parts, as this will increase your metabolic rate, leading to an increase in blood flow and an over-reaction in the inflammatory process.

Ice

Ice minimises bleeding, swelling and pain. It should be applied immediately by placing a damp towel containing chipped or crushed ice (use cold water if no ice is available) over or around the injury. Apply for 10 to 30 minutes every 2 hours. If you have very low body fat, do not apply ice or cold for more than 10 minutes. Never return to activity immediately following the application of ice or cold. Ice burns and nerve damage can occur from applying ice incorrectly.

Compression

If you can see any swelling (remember it may increase), apply a compression bandage

- a minimum of 15 cm above and below the injury;
- in a spiral fashion – not around the limb;
- from distal (far) to proximal (near) (e.g., from ankle to hip or wrist to shoulder); and
- for injuries in the hand or foot, level with the webs of the fingers or toes.

Do not overstretch the bandage. The compression must be firm but not so tight as to cause discomfort. Pressure must be even throughout, *not* greater at one end. Remove and reapply the bandage if uniform and constant pressure is not maintained. Use protective padding to protect vulnerable areas (e.g., inside of the elbow). Check the fingers or toes regularly; if they are cold or pale, the compression is too tight.

Elevation

Raise the injured part above the level of the heart as soon as possible after injury and as often as possible for the first 3 days following injury. Support the injured part on pillows or in a sling. If the limb can be maintained in elevation, you need not apply compression at the same time. To avoid swelling after elevation, apply compression prior to lowering the injured limb.

Even if you are satisfied with your progress, talk to a doctor or chartered physiotherapist to check that you are doing everything possible to return quickly and safely to your sport, without the chance of a recurrence.

Rehabilitation

Do you know what to do to help you recover as quickly and safely as possible? After prevention and immediate treatment, you need to think about the injury rehabilitation process – how to resume your sport as quickly and safely as possible. The rehabilitation phase includes the

- later stages of treatment and rehabilitation,
- testing for fitness after injury, and
- returning to training and competition.

Further Treatment

For first- and second-degree soft tissue injuries, the inflammatory process changes between day 3 and day 10, and you may gradually start exercising to regain joint and muscle mobility and muscle endurance. If necessary, you can apply gentle heat and massage around (not over) the injured area. It is very important that any massage, exercises or any other treatment you receive does not increase pain or discomfort. If you experience any discomfort or pain, tell the person treating you because he or she may wish to adjust the treatment.

In the later stages of treatment or rehabilitation, from day 11 onwards, the emphasis is on regaining

- full mobility of all relevant joints and muscles;
- full endurance in all the muscles that may have been affected by the injury;
- full strength in all the muscles that may have been affected by the injury;
- full power or speed in all the muscles that may have been affected by the injury;
- balance, especially when practising the skills of your sport; and
- your previous skill level.

If you have injured an arm or leg, you can compare the injured limb with the opposite limb to judge how your recovery is progressing. Although it is important to regain all the components of fitness listed above, the process cannot be rushed. Your body can heal only at a certain rate. You are trying to provide the best environment for healing to take place. If you try to rush any of the stages, you will often delay, or even reverse, the healing process.

> The healing process cannot be rushed. Your body recovers at a set rate. Trying to rush any of the stages of healing often results in delay.

Fitness Testing

Following injury, testing for fitness is an important part of the treatment programme. Such testing is made up of small steps that show how you are progressing. For example, you should not suddenly sprint if you have not practised jogging, running at half pace, then three-quarter pace, gradually increasing your acceleration and deceleration. Progress must be made slowly and not viewed as some sort of competition. It allows you, your coach and all the support staff to know whether it is safe for you to return to modified training, full training and finally to competition.

Full Recovery

Return to training and competition should occur only when you and everyone concerned with your treatment and fitness are completely satisfied that you

- have fully regained the components of fitness;

- have regained your previous aerobic and anaerobic fitness, which you may have lost while you were unable to train;
- have recovered your skill level and co-ordination; and
- are match fit.

Sports Massage

Do you know the benefits of sports massage? Massage, which has a long tradition of use within sport, is a mechanical manipulation of the body's tissues using rhythmical pressure and stroking and is used to promote health and well-being.

Massage is said to

- increase the blood flow and delivery of oxygen,
- improve the transfer of nutrients and waste products in the capillaries,
- improve the drainage of tissue fluid into the veins and lymph vessels,
- decrease or remove lactic acid from the muscles after exercise,
- help remove the substances that cause pain, and
- improve your sense of well-being.

Athletes believe massage improves performance and aids recovery. This may be true because it has a local heating effect on the blood vessels, causing them to dilate (widen) and increasing the blood flow without increasing metabolism (cell energy). It causes a change in pressure, which encourages blood to be carried through the capillaries, where the transfer of nutrients and waste products takes place. It is *not* an effective substitute for warm-up or cool-down and has little effect on flexibility. However, it may help endurance exercises by increasing muscle blood flow, delivery of oxygen and muscle temperature.

It can also have a psychological effect by improving the mood of the performer.

Athletes use massage, therefore, to

- prepare for training and competition,
- recover from training and competition, and
- treat injuries.

When getting a massage, keep in mind that it should be given in a warm environment and the body should be covered. A massage should not cause discomfort or pain; overly vigorous massage may damage muscle and other soft tissue. Finally, massage should not be given near an injury that is less than 3 days old or in an area where there is an infection.

Assessing Your Needs

To help you assess your attitudes towards your health and to injuries, complete Task 28. This assessment will also provide you with a profile score out of 10 for each component (refer back to the self-profiling exercise you did beginning on page 11).

Task 28	Assessing Your Attitudes Towards Health and Injuries

Based on the advice in this chapter, rate yourself on each of the following using the 10-point scale (1 = very poor, 10 = could not be better)

Measures you take to look after your health	1 2 3 4 5 6 7 8 9 10
Ability to stay injury-free	1 2 3 4 5 6 7 8 9 10
Measures you take to avoid injuries	1 2 3 4 5 6 7 8 9 10
Actions you take when injured	1 2 3 4 5 6 7 8 9 10
Attitude during rehabilitation	1 2 3 4 5 6 7 8 9 10

Identify what you would like to improve most and how you might go about it:

Key Points

- Record your resting heart rate to find out how your body is coping with training. Any decreases in your heart rate show that you're becoming more fit, whereas increases are a warning sign that the body is not coping with the training load.
- Be aware of potential injury risks. Identifying these risks can help you to avoid injury.
- Use the PRICE guide (Protection, Rest, Ice, Compression, Elevation) to treat first- and second-degree soft tissue injuries, or as a first-aid device before you seek professional advice.
- Always seek advice from professionals if you have second- or third-degree injuries.

Getting Serious

Always remember why you take part in sport. As someone who is performance oriented you should be serious about what you do, but that doesn't mean you should not continue to have fun.

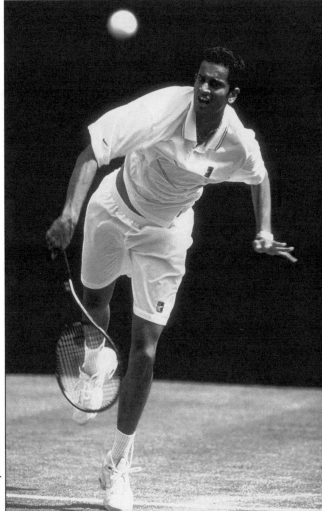

Courtesy of Nike, Inc.

In this part, you will find information on topics that may not be relevant to all young athletes immediately. It should therefore be used for reference when the need arises.

The first chapter is on training and competing abroad, although it contains plenty of advice that will prove equally useful to anyone travelling abroad for holiday or business purposes. Increasingly, athletes of all levels are travelling abroad for training camps and competitions. As an elite athlete, you may have already experienced this and will know some of the difficulties you may encounter: changes in weather, time zones, food and culture, to name but a few. Overseas training and competitions can provide great experience, but they can also be disastrous if you do not take advice and plan well in advance. Chapter 7 will help you to do this so you can enjoy the experience and benefit fully from it.

Chapter 8 on drugs and testing should be read by any elite athlete, for you need to be aware of drugs – the dangers of the illegal and so-called performance-enhancing drugs, as well as the problems with over-the-counter medicines that may contain banned substances. You may at some stage be subject to drug testing, and this can be quite unnerving, especially the first time. This chapter tries to dispel the myths about drugs and provide clear advice on how to check any medicines you take and how to cope with the drug-testing procedure.

CHAPTER 7

Training and Competing Abroad

As an elite athlete, or someone aspiring to that level, you are likely to be involved in training and competing abroad, and this often means you need to adjust to different environments, lifestyles and time zones. In Great Britain, you live at or near sea level, in a fairly cool climate, but you may find yourself at a training camp or competition where it is much hotter and more humid and perhaps even at a high altitude. The food will be different, the water may or may not be fit to drink and your body will be vulnerable to a new range of potential illnesses. Therefore, it is important to know what to do to ensure you can perform your very best. In this chapter, you will find general travel tips, as well as specific advice on the following:

1. Flying right
2. Adjusting to different time zones
3. Travelling smart

There are no tasks in this chapter, as it is meant to be more of a reference point for you.

Flying Right

The hassle associated with checking in and out of airports and passing through customs can cause a general sense of fatigue. This will often be increased by having to lose sleep as a result of the time spent on your journey or a change in time zones. Another problem is caused by the air in the plane, which tends to cause dehydration and headaches, and the lack of movement that is possible during flight can lead to stiffness and even cramping. However, you can do several things to counteract these potential problems.

First, drink plenty of water (take some with you), fruit juice, squashes and still mineral waters. Coffee, tea and alcohol are likely to be offered on the flight, but these are diuretics, so don't drink too much of them. This is not meant as deprivation, but an attempt to guard against the dehydration produced by the dry air in the cabin.

Many convenience foods are low in fibre (roughage) and might cause constipation. Try to eat foods that are high in roughage, such as fresh fruit, whole-grain bread or rolls, celery or carrots. You might want to take along some sandwiches or snacks to make sure you have something you like. You don't have to eat everything that is provided.

Try to take some exercise during the flight (not a full workout) to decrease stiffness and the possibility of cramping. A few stretches may also be done in the aisle or out of sight at the back of the cabin, or a stroll down the aisle may be sufficient.

Keep active during the flight by walking about and stretching.

Set your watch to the arrival time zone immediately after take-off. During the flight, try to sleep if it is nighttime at your destination; when it is daytime there, try to stay awake by finding somebody to talk to, reading a book or watching the in-flight movie.

Adjusting to Different Time Zones

Countries have a local time that is fixed by the position of the earth in relation to the sun. For example, when it is 4 P.M. in England, it is 11 A.M. in New York, but 8 P.M. in Abu Dhabi and midnight in Singapore. As you travel from one country to another, you often cross time zones and have to adjust to new times. This disturbs your internal body clock. Jet-lag refers to a number of symptoms caused by such disturbances and seems to affect travellers in different ways and to different extents. Fortunately, people who are younger and more fit tend to suffer far less from its negative effects. The symptoms include fatigue, inability to sleep at the right time, loss of appetite, constipation, loss of concentration and motivation and headaches.

Although jet-lag affects individuals differently, generally it is more severe and lasts longer after a flight to the east and becomes more pronounced the more time zones you cross.

Several psychological and physiological factors are influenced by your internal clock. Alertness and sleepiness are good examples. If you do not go to sleep at the usual time, you start to feel tired as the night progresses. If you stay up long enough, from about 5 A.M. onwards you will begin to feel more wide awake in spite of having had no sleep. This is your internal clock waking you up for a new day.

It is no surprise to learn that world records are not broken in the middle of the night. However, that is exactly the problem for an athlete who has just flown across several time zones and must compete at a time that corresponds to his normal nighttime. Full adjustment of the body clock takes several days, although you can start the adjustment process during the flight and even before travelling.

You can do this by starting to adjust your lifestyle to the new time zone in the days immediately before departure. One possibility if flying west, where time is behind the UK, is to go to bed 1 to 2 hours later than normal each night and get up 1 to 2 hours later each morning. In contrast, if flying east, where time is ahead of the UK, try going to bed 1 to 2 hours earlier each night and getting up 1 to 2 hours earlier each day. You will find it difficult to make any further adjustments, as it will start to interfere too much with your training schedule and lifestyle. On the plane, remember to try to sleep if it is nighttime at your destination and to stay awake when it is daytime there.

On arrival, make sure you stick to the new time zone and avoid the temptation of working out the time back home. If you wake early (often because you need to pass urine), return quietly to bed until the correct rising time. Similarly, even if you do not feel like going to bed at your normal bedtime, you should do so and lie quietly and relax. If you feel tired during the day, resist the temptation to take a nap unless genuinely exhausted from lack of sleep.

Even though you won't feel like tackling a full training session at first, light exercise out of doors and brisk walks taken at your accustomed time in the local time zone will help you adjust to the new time and make you feel ready for sleep at bedtime. Try to take meals of the correct type (i.e., breakfast, lunch) at the appropriate time. Do not eat a large supper that may make sleep difficult.

If you have to compete soon after arriving in a new time zone and before you have fully recovered from your jet-lag, you should adopt the new and

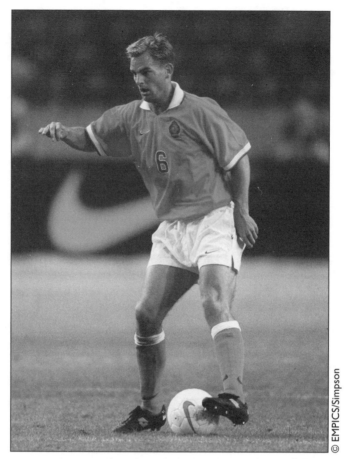

Elite athletes can help themselves stay sharp and focused when competing abroad by adjusting to the new time zone a few days before they leave.

regular regime of sleep, activity and meals as much as possible. It may also be a good idea to take a short nap before an important event but rise at least 2 hours before it.

Travelling Smart

The following tips make good sense whether you are travelling for your sport or simply on holiday.

Well before you go,

- make sure your passport is up to date (make a separate note of the number in case of loss) and check whether you need a visa;
- check with your doctor whether you need any immunisations;
- have a dental check;

- organise some local currency;
- arrange a BT charge card so you have a cheap way to call home;
- find out about the voltage and power points and buy an adapter as necessary; and
- buy any special foods you want to take with you (e.g., British tea or a certain breakfast cereal).

When travelling,

- always carry your important competition equipment and shoes with you on the flight;
- wear loose, comfortable clothes;
- leave plenty of time to check in at the airport; and
- remember to take some snacks and water with you.

On arrival,

- do not take risks if you are unsure about the level of sanitation; if you have any concerns:
  a. do not eat unwashed food;
  b. use bottled water for drinking and cleaning your teeth;
  c. do not have ice in your drinks;
  d. eat only in well-known or recommended places; and
  e. avoid seafood, spicy food and other food you do not usually eat.
- respect local customs.
- remember to keep drinking small amounts and often, especially if it is hot.

Key Points

- During the flight, drink plenty of fluids to avoid dehydration (avoid alcohol and caffeine), and try to stretch or exercise to avoid stiffness.
- Adjust to a new time zone a few days before you leave and keep to that new time zone once you've arrived.
- Carry important competition equipment with you on the flight.

The information in this chapter was written by Sarah Rowell with information supplied by the British Olympic Association.

Understanding Drugs and Doping

You will no doubt have heard stories about competitors using drugs and doping in an attempt to improve their performance. To reach the top in any sport requires talent, hard work and dedication. If you use performance-enhancing drugs and doping methods, you are cheating. Cheating not only affects your fellow competitors, but also yourself, your health, your supporters and your sport. This chapter is divided into the following two sections:

1. Doping methods
2. Doping control

Doping Methods

A drug is any substance that affects your emotional state, body function or behaviour. Drugs include alcohol, tobacco, caffeine, anabolic steroids and all over-the-counter medications. They may be either harmful or beneficial, and you should be aware of the following categories of drugs:

- **Social drugs** (so called), which are often classified into soft drugs such as cannabis and hard drugs such as heroin, cocaine and crack. The Misuse of Drugs Act (1971) controls both hard and soft drugs, and it is a criminal offence to supply or possess these substances. Some athletes are fooled by the myth that taking some forms of illegal drugs will help them relax and therefore will help them to perform better. Usually, however, taking such substances makes your performance worse.

- **Performance-enhancing drugs** (e.g., anabolic steroids and peptide hormones) are taken by some performers in an attempt to improve their performance or the way their bodies look. However, taking such drugs is against the rules of the International Olympic Committee (IOC) and most governing bodies of sport. Different types of performance-enhancing drugs will be considered in more detail later.

- **Medications** (e.g., cough and cold medicines and painkillers) are designed to treat illness and injury. As a competitor, you need to know that there are some common over-the-counter medications you should not take, as they contain performance-enhancing substances and are therefore not allowed in sport (e.g., Sudafed and Lemsip powder).

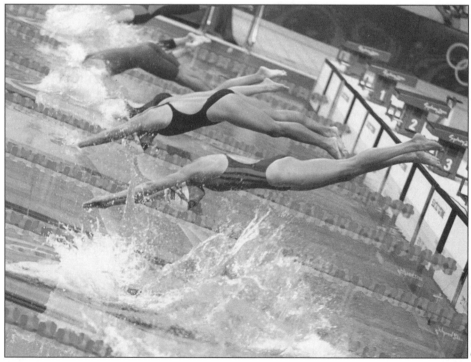

© EMPICS/Buckle

All athletes should be aware of what is in any medication they're taking to ensure it doesn't contain banned substances that could keep them out of competition.

Even when taking permitted medications such as non-steroidal anti-inflammatory painkillers, you should remember never to misuse them. Continuing to compete or train while injured or ill usually results in the problem's getting worse and lasting longer, rather than getting better.

• **Nutritional supplements** are frequently promoted as having an ergogenic or performance-enhancing effect. Most of these products contain only vitamins, minerals and natural herbal extracts. However, as they are not subject to stringent licensing, their content and status cannot be determined. Some, for example, contain banned substances (e.g., Guarana, Ma Huang and Chinese Ephedra). Before taking any such product, you should always make sure you read the ingredients label very carefully and understand what all the substances listed are. If you are in any doubt, do not take the product. Remember, just because someone else is taking it does not mean it is safe to do so.

Performance-Enhancing Substances

In this section, you will find more information on various types of banned drugs and doping methods, including examples of banned drugs, details of the health risks and some reasons why performers have been tempted to take them. Because it is not possible to list all the substances and medications that are either prohibited or allowed in each category, it is strongly recommended that you obtain a copy of the publication *Competitors and Officials Guide to Drugs and Sport*, which can be obtained from UK Sport at a cost of £6.00.

Stimulants

Stimulants act on the brain and are banned, as they can provide performers with an unfair physical and mental advantage by reducing tiredness and increasing competitiveness, alertness and aggression.

Harmful side effects include

• a rise in blood pressure and body temperature,
• an increased and irregular heartbeat,
• aggressiveness and anxiety,
• loss of appetite, and
• addiction.

Performers have died from misuse of stimulants, as they make it difficult for the body to cool down, resulting in dehydration and ultimately failure of the circulatory system. Examples of stimulants include amphetamine, phentermine, cocaine, diethylpropion, ephedrine, caffeine (or Guarana) and phenylpropanolamine. Be aware that ephedrine and phenylpropanolamine are often found in low doses in some cough and cold medications.

You may be surprised that caffeine is listed as a stimulant and is therefore a banned drug. However, this does not mean you cannot have any products that contain caffeine. Allowed products include tea, coffee, cola, chocolate, Feminax, Pro-plus, Red Bull or Red Kick, Panadol Extra or Hedex Extra. Caffeine ingestion has been shown to increase endurance and power in many sports. It is also a diuretic (i.e., increases urine output). For this reason, caffeine is considered a prohibited substance at concentrations above 12 micrograms per millilitre of urine. If you have a normal caffeine intake, you should not reach this level. To reach the prohibited level, you would need to drink approximately 3 to 10 cups of coffee or tea (depending on the brand and brewing method) or 9 cans of soft drink in a short time period and be tested soon after drinking them. These are approximations only, as the concentration of caffeine in the sample will depend on a range of individual variations (e.g., your weight, metabolic rate and what you have eaten recently will all have an effect on the level of caffeine in your body, so care is required). You should, therefore, be aware of all the sources of caffeine that you take and the amount of caffeine in each product. For example, the amount of caffeine in a cup of tea will increase the longer the bag is infused in the cup or pot.

Narcotic Analgesics

Narcotic analgesics are painkillers that act on the brain to reduce the amount of pain felt. Performers use them illegally to reduce pain (e.g., from injuries or illness), increase their pain threshold or hide injuries. Harmful side effects include

- further damage to the original injury;
- breathing problems, nausea and vomiting;
- loss of concentration, balance and co-ordination; and
- addiction.

Examples of narcotic analgesics that are prohibited include methadone, morphine and pethidine. Aspirin, paracetamol and dihydrocodeine are allowed.

Androgenic Anabolic Steroids

Androgenic anabolic steroids (also known as anabolic steroids) are a type of hormone that includes testosterone and substances with a similar chemical structure and effect. They are used by competitors to increase muscle size and strength and to increase aggression, which in turn may help athletes to train harder. Androgenic anabolic steroids affect people in different ways, as they interfere with the body's normal hormone balance.

Anyone taking steroids is at increased risk of

- liver disease,
- premature heart disease,
- increased aggression, and
- infectious diseases (such as HIV and hepatitis) if taken by injection.

Males taking steroids can suffer from

- acne,
- kidney damage,
- development of breasts,
- premature baldness, and
- shrinking and hardening of the testicles.

Females taking steroids can suffer from

- the development of male features, including deepening of the voice;
- irregular periods; and
- increased body hair growth.

Adolescents taking steroids can suffer from

- stunted growth and
- severe acne on the face and body.

Anabolic steroids bought on the black market may be fakes or may contain impurities that can cause serious and sometimes fatal side effects. Examples of anabolic steroids include boldenone, mesterolone, methandienone, testosterone, nandrolone and stanozolol.

Beta-Blockers

Beta-blockers are banned in some sports, so you should check with your governing body medical officer. They lower the heart rate and blood pressure and are used by doctors to treat heart disease. Competitors misuse them in an attempt to steady their nerves and to stop trembling, particularly in sports requiring fine muscular control and calmness, such as shooting and archery.

Harmful side effects include

- low blood pressure,
- reduced heart rate, and
- tiredness.

Examples of beta-blockers include atenolol, oxprenolol and propranolol.

Diuretics

Diuretics help remove fluid from the body. Competitors may misuse them either to

- reduce weight quickly (e.g., in sports with weight categories such as judo and boxing) or
- as a masking agent; the increased urine makes it more difficult for a laboratory to detect other banned substances such as anabolic steroids.

Abuse of diuretics can cause

- dehydration,
- faintness and dizziness,
- muscle cramps, and
- headaches and nausea.

Examples of diuretics include bendrofluazide, triamterine, frusemide, spironolactone and hydrochlorothiazide.

Peptide Hormones and Mimetics

Peptide hormones and mimetics* are taken by performers to stimulate the production of naturally occurring steroids, build muscle, enhance body healing and increase the body's ability to carry oxygen. Peptide hormones are secreted by the body, for example, to increase growth, control pain and influence sexual and general behaviour. The mimetics have a similar effect, but it is difficult to know how much harm misuse of these can cause.

Examples of peptide hormones and mimetics include the following:

- Chorionic gonadotrophin (HCG): In males this drug has a similar effect to using testosterone.
- Corticotrophin (ACTH): This drug helps repair damaged tissues, including muscles, but may cause muscle wasting if used for long periods of time.
- Growth hormone (HGH): If used to increase muscle size, there is a risk of abnormal growth of the hands, feet, face and internal organs, including the liver.
- Erythropoietin (EPO): This drug has a similar effect to blood doping in that it increases the number of red blood cells. This thickening of the blood can be dangerous, leading to clots or overloading the heart and increased risk of suffering from a stroke.

---

*Mimetics or analogues are man-made (synthetic) drugs that affect the body in a similar way to hormones.

- Insulin: This drug is permitted only for treating insulin-dependent diabetes. Written notification of insulin-dependent diabetes is required.

Blood Doping

Blood doping is the injection of blood into an athlete's body to increase the number of red blood cells. This practice increases the amount of oxygen the blood can carry to the working muscles during exercise and so helps improve performance. EPO has a similar effect. Harmful side effects of blood doping include

- allergic reactions,
- hepatitis or AIDS,
- overload of the circulatory system, and
- blood clots and kidney damage.

Safe Medication

The preceding section gave examples of prohibited substances, but there are many medications that are permitted; examples are listed in table 8.1.

Before taking any over-the-counter medications or medicines prescribed by your GP, always remember to check the label or ask the doctor or pharmacist whether the product is suitable for an elite athlete.

Doping Control

International and national sports organisations have introduced a doping control process to catch those who misuse drugs or use doping methods and to deter performers from misusing drugs. These organisations also help raise awareness about the potential dangers to a competitor's health through drug misuse. This is all done in an effort to preserve and maintain the ethics and values of sport.

If you are an elite competitor in the UK, it is likely that you will come into contact with the drug-testing programme operated by UK Sport. This programme and the one run by your sport's international federation may mean that you could be required to provide a urine sample for testing at major national or international competitions. You may also be tested during training or, if your sport has an out-of-competition testing programme, at your place of study, work or home. Although each sport may have slightly different rules about doping, the basic principles of the testing procedures used to collect urine samples are similar.

Table 8.1 Permissible Drugs

Illness or condition	Permitted treatment
Asthma	Sodium cromoglycate, theophylline, salbutamol*, terbutaline*, salmeterol*, beclomethasone**, fluticasone**
Cold or cough	All antibiotics, steam and menthol inhalers, paracetamol, permitted antihistamines, terfenadine, astemizole, pholcodine, guaphenesin, dextromethorphan
Diarrhoea	Diphenoxylate, loperamide, products containing electrolytes (i.e., Dioralyte and Rehidrat)
Hay fever	Permitted antihistamines, nasal sprays containing a corticosteroid or xylometazoline, eyedrops containing sodium cromoglycate
Pain	Aspirin, codeine, dihydrocodeine, ibuprofen, paracetamol, all non-steroidal anti-inflammatories, dextropropoxyphene
Vomiting	Domperidone, metoclopramide

*These can be taken only by inhalation and only following written notification to your national governing body.

**Permitted by inhalation; check with your governing body whether notification is required.

The drug-testing procedure is described in the following steps, based on various publications produced by the UK Sport Ethics and Anti-Doping Directorate.

It is a good idea to familiarise yourself with this process before being called for drug testing. Remember, you are allowed to have a representative of your choice present during the whole of the testing procedure, apart from in the toilet, when you provide the sample. Therefore, you may wish to have a parent or guardian, coach or team manager present, particularly if you have never been drug tested before.

The following paragraphs describe the drug-testing process:

1. **Notification.** You will be given written notice by a UK Sport Independent Sampling Officer (ISO) if you have been selected for a drug test. At this point, you will be asked to sign the form acknowledging you have been advised of your rights and have received the notice. If you are selected for out-of-competition testing, you may be given little or no notice of the test. If the ISO contacts you first by phone, you will need to meet the ISO as soon as possible to provide a sample. You will be asked to sign a notification form at the testing session.

2. **Providing the sample.** You will accompany the ISO to the Doping Control Station or, if out-of-competition testing, a suitable private venue where sealed non-alcoholic, caffeine-free drinks should be available. When you are ready to provide a urine sample, you will be asked to select a sealed collection vessel and go to the toilet with the ISO. When providing the urine sample, you must do so under the direct supervision of the ISO, having removed sufficient clothes so the ISO can see you giving the sample.

3. **Sealed bottles.** You will then be asked by the ISO to select a sealed urine sampling kit. Make sure you check that the security seal is intact. If satisfied, open the kit. The kit will contain two bottles: A and B. You will be asked to divide your sample between the two bottles and to seal them tightly. A few drops of your urine sample need to be left in the collection vessel so that pH and specific gravity can be tested. The ISO will then invite you to check that the two bottles are properly sealed and that there is no leakage. It is important to check this.

4. **Initial tests.** Next the ISO will check the pH and specific gravity of your urine sample. The pH test measures the degree of acidity or alkalinity of the sample, and the specific gravity test ensures that it is not too diluted. All samples collected are sent to the laboratory for testing, even if the pH or specific gravity are outside the normal limits. If this is the case, it will be recorded on the sample collection form, and you will be asked to provide a second sample. Refusing to give a second sample may be considered as a failure to agree with the request for testing and may be treated in the same way as a positive drug test.

5. **Labelling**. The ISO will write the sample numbers on the sample collection form. Make sure you check that this information is correct. You will also be asked for details of any drugs or medications that you have taken during the last 7 days. Although you do not have to give this information, it is much better to record anything you have taken, even if you do not think it is a drug (e.g., treatment for a cold).

6. **Confirmation.** Finally, the ISO will ask you and your representative to check that all the information recorded on the sample collection form is correct. If you agree with what is recorded, you will be asked to sign the form. The ISO will also check and sign the form.

7. **Lab testing.** Your sample will then go in a sealed bag for testing at an IOC-accredited laboratory.

8. **Negative results.** If the analysis of the A sample is negative, UK Sport will be informed of the result within 10 days of the test and the B sample will be destroyed.

9. **Positive results.** If the A sample gives a positive result, you will be offered the opportunity to have the B sample analysed. If the results

from this are also positive, the findings will be passed to your governing body disciplinary panel.

Other useful publications available from the UK Sport Ethics and Anti-Doping Directorate include

- *Drug Testing Procedures* – a guide for competitors and officials (free),
- *Doping Classes and Methods* – a free advice card, and
- *Competitors and Officials Guide to Drugs and Sport* – a comprehensive drugs and sport publication written for athletes (cost, £6.00)

For further information on the drug-testing process, contact the Anti-Doping Directorate by phone on 0270 380 8030 or by e-mail at ethicsanti.doping@uksport.gov.uk.

Key Points

- You need to be aware of various types of drugs and the effects they have on the body.
- Before taking any over-the-counter medicines, check with the doctor or pharmacist to see if the product is suitable for an elite athlete.
- If in doubt about any medication, check with your governing body medical officer or UK Sport's Ethics and Anti-Doping Directorate (0270 380 8030) or **drug.enquiries@uksport.gov.uk**.
- Familiarise yourself with the process of doping control. Have a parent or guardian, coach or team manager present the first time you are tested.

The information in this chapter was written by Sarah Rowell with information from various publications produced by UK Sport Ethics and Anti-Doping Directorate. For more information, contact the Directorate by telephone on 0270 380 8030 or by e-mail at ethicsanti.doping@uksport.gov.uk, © UK Sport.

PART IV

Planning for Success

Plan and be patient. Reaching the top in any sport takes time and may seem like it is a long way off. You can make it easier by setting reachable targets as stepping stones toward your ultimate goal.

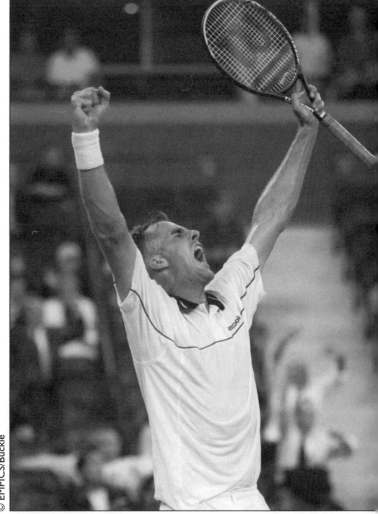

In this final part, you can put into practice all the guidance and new ideas you have gained from reading this performance pack. For this reason, you need to work through this part last.

In chapter 9, you will have a chance to re-profile yourself. You will now be able to do a more detailed profile because you will have examined several factors more closely: the specific fitness requirements of your sport, the importance of food and fluids, the way mental skills can improve your sport performance and what you can do to stay healthy and injury-free. After that, you will be able to set more specific goals for the forthcoming season and plan your competitions and training, as well as everything else that is important to keep your life balanced and you happy.

In the final chapter, you will learn some ways to help you put your plan into practice and monitor your progress towards your goals. You will be able to design your own training diary to help you plan and monitor your own pathway to success.

CHAPTER 9

Putting It All Together

Now that you have worked through the performance pack, you can put it all together and ensure that you really do train smarter by working on quality training focused on the areas most important to success for you and for your sport. In this chapter, you can re-work your performance profile to identify your priority areas and your goals for the forthcoming season. You can then map out your programme for the year, identifying training phases, key competitions and training camps, as well as important dates at school, for the family and with friends. You will then be in a good position to break down your season's goals into shorter-term goals and start to plot your training.

This chapter is divided into two sections:

1. Profiling and action planning
2. Creating a yearly planner

Profiling and Action Planning

Having worked through this pack, you are now in a position to compile a more informed and probably more specific performance profile. The best time to do this is during the recovery phase, but if you are in the pre- or early-season phases, it is well worth working through the planning.

Start by looking back on your analysis of your sport (pages 5-8); you may find you want to make a few adjustments. Then study your own performance profile (pages 11-15) and the more specific profile attributes you rated in the chapters on fitness (pages 38, 45, 49 and 60), nutrition (page 75), mental skills (pages 90 and 96) and health and injury (page 108). Having done this, you can tackle Task 29.

Task 29 Creating a More Specific Performance Profile

1. Think of the ideal athlete in your sport; it may help to think of the highly successful athletes and the ones you admire. Write down the attributes that would describe this ideal athlete.

   Skills (e.g., technical/tactical, personal, mental): _____

   _____

   _____

   _____

   Knowledge (e.g., of sport, training, world practice, competition, nutrition and supplements, injury management): _____

   _____

   _____

   _____

   Attitudes (e.g., towards other athletes, coaches or officials; towards success and failure; towards injury management, training, competition, financial gain and sponsorship, career and life outside sport): _____

   _____

   _____

   _____

2. Now select and describe 10 attributes you feel are the most important for success in your sport and write these in the following appropriate columns. Try to be quite specific; for example, don't just write *fitness,* but specify which component of fitness is important for your sport and for you.

Attributes	Description	Rating
1.		1 2 3 4 5 6 7 8 9 10
2.		1 2 3 4 5 6 7 8 9 10
3.		1 2 3 4 5 6 7 8 9 10
4.		1 2 3 4 5 6 7 8 9 10
5.		1 2 3 4 5 6 7 8 9 10
6.		1 2 3 4 5 6 7 8 9 10
7.		1 2 3 4 5 6 7 8 9 10
8.		1 2 3 4 5 6 7 8 9 00
9.		1 2 3 4 5 6 7 8 9 10
10.		1 2 3 4 5 6 7 8 9 10

3. Next rate yourself (this should be your opinion, no guidance from your coach, teacher or anyone else) honestly on the 10-point scale (1 = very poor and 10 = could not be better). When rating yourself, think of the athlete you want to become (i.e., few, if any, 10s); leave room for improvement. It may help to look back at some of the ratings you gave yourself for particular attributes in each chapter.

(continued)

Task 29 *(continued)*

4. Transfer the attributes and your rating onto the circular profile that follows:

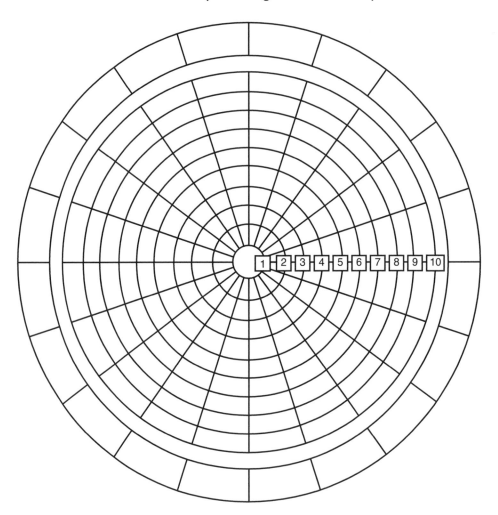

5. Next decide where you would like to be on each attribute by the end of the season (or 12 months' time). Be realistic (you can't expect to make big differences on each one), but give yourself a challenge. You may want to prioritise and go for a bigger improvement on those attributes you feel would have a significant positive impact on your performance. Mark the segment on the score you want to attain. Refer back to page 15 if you need a reminder of how to do this.

6. Write down your main goals for the next year; some of these may be outcome goals, some may be performance goals, but they should be SMART goals (refer back to page 84, if necessary). They may relate to sport, school or any important aspect of your life during the next 12 months. Where

appropriate, they should relate directly or indirectly to your profiled attribute, and where possible, try to ensure that you have a balance between technical, tactical, personal, fitness, mental and so on. Use the prompts in the next box, or if they do not help, use a blank sheet of paper.

Season's goals:

Goals for sport (e.g., selection, result, time, score):

Outcome/performance/process goals (technical, tactical): _____

_____

_____

Outcome/performance/process goals (fitness, nutrition, health): _____

_____

_____

Outcome/performance/process goals (mental, personal): _____

_____

_____

Goals outside sport (e.g., academic, social, family):

Outcome/performance/process goals (academic, school, work): _____

_____

_____

Outcome/performance/process goals (home): _____

_____

_____

Outcome/performance/process goals (social): _____

_____

_____

Outcome/performance/process goals (other): _____

_____

_____

7. It would be a good idea to share these with relevant members of *Team You* (your coach and perhaps your parent or guardian and/or teacher) before continuing.

Creating a Yearly Planner

Before breaking down these seasonal goals into shorter-term goals and more specific action plans, it is important to look more closely at the forthcoming year. You will complete a yearly planner, but before attempting this, you will need to find answers to the questions in Task 30 (you may need to ask your coach, teacher or parent or guardian to help with some sections).

Task 30	Identifying Important Dates in the Forthcoming Year

1. This is my planner for the year _____

2. My main sport for the year is _____

3. My main team/club for the year is _____

4. Team/club selection takes place on _____

5. County/regional team/squad selection is on _____

6. National team/squad selection is on _____

7. Other sports teams/squads I am involved with _____

   _____

8. My coaches are _____ (main) and

   _____ (others)

9. Members of *Team You* include _____

   _____

10. Key competition/match dates for the year (e.g., club championships 3/3/01)

    _____

11. Key academic dates for the year (e.g., year exams 26/12/01; GCSE mocks 21/3/01) _____

12. Family and other social dates (e.g., 1 week in Majorca 7-14 September)

    _____

    _____

    _____

    _____

You can now create an annual planner by following the steps in Task 31.

It is very important to plan your year to ensure you are at your best when it really matters.

Task 31 Completing a Training Planner

1. Use the planner in figure 9.3 to plot the most important events in the year (competitions, overseas training camps, school exams, family occasions, special events). Note when you want to be at your very best and identify any hot spots. You will need to resolve these with your coach, parent or guardian and/or teacher before you can continue with this task. See the sample training planner in figure 9.2 for help.

2. Next ask your coach to help you complete the section on training intensity and type by identifying the different types of fitness and training work you will be doing throughout the year. You will need to use a different line for each type of training and identify the intensity of the training by marking the row at the top (high intensity) or at the bottom (low intensity); see the sample training planner in figure 9.2 for help.

Note: When completing the training intensity and type, remember to take into account your school, family and other social commitments (e.g., you may not want to do a lot of training when you are on holiday or when taking exams).

Training planner for the year beginning: _____

Hot spots					X
Month (write in the months)	1 Sep.	2 Oct.	3 Nov.	4 Dec.	5 Jan.
Most important **Competitions** (place most important competitions where you want peak performance at the top of the column, less important ones toward the bottom) Least important			Club champs. 3/3/00	County trials	County comp.
Academic and social					GCSE mocks
Training intensity and type (see note in instructions)	High — Aerobic Strength Skills and tactics — Low				

Figure 9.2 Sample training planner.

	X					
6 Feb.	7 Mar.	8 Apr.	9 May	10 June	11 July	12 Aug.

National comp.

Intl. comp.

Intl. tour

End-of-year course work

Holiday!

Training planner for the year beginning: _____

Hot spots					
Month (write in the months)					
Most important **Competitions** (place most important competitions where you want peak performance at the top of the column, less important ones toward the bottom) Least important					
Academic and social					
High **Training intensity and type** (see note in instructions) Low					

Figure 9.3 Create your own training planner using this blank form.

Now that you have mapped out your training plan and determined your seasonal goals, you can begin to break down your seasonal goals into shorter-term goals and more specific action plans. Task 32 provides a few sample goals to help you get started.

Task 32 Completing Your Goals and Action Plans

Seasonal goal	Shorter-term goals (with dates)	How I will achieve (specific actions to take)	Progress against goals and action steps
To gain selection for the under-18 county netball squad (February)	To develop my pre-shooting imagery routine and use it 100% of the time (September)	Develop the routine and work on it at home five times a week (August)	
		Try the routine in every training session and adapt it as necessary (September)	
		Use the routine in competition (from September)	
	To improve my power test rating by 5% (November tests)	Work on maximum strength of legs in weights and circuit work in preseason phase	
		Do two plyometric sessions a week (early season)	
		Maintain strength and power work with two weights/circuit sessions a week throughout season	
	To increase my shooting percentage from 70 to 85% in competitions (December)	Fix goalpost at home so I can do 5 x 20-min. technical shooting sessions a week throughout pre- and early-season	
		Log shooting percentage in training (early and preseason)	
		Log shooting percentage in matches (throughout season)	

Seasonal goal	Shorter-term goals (with dates)	How I will achieve (specific actions to take)	Progress against goals and action steps

Don't forget to share your goal setting and action planning with *Team You*, especially your coach (and parent or guardian, when appropriate). In addition to placing a copy of your goals in your diary, it is a good idea to display them in a place where you will see them regularly (perhaps in your bedroom, at your desk or beside your mirror).

Key Points

- Create your own annual training planner by identifying important dates in the forthcoming year.
- Plan your year and set goals to ensure that you're at your best when it matters most.

CHAPTER 10

Designing a Training Diary

Finally, to make the whole planning exercise a success, you need to develop a system that will help you plan, chart, record and monitor your progress against your goals.

Most elite athletes use some form of a training log or diary. Although this may seem like a chore, it is

- essential to be systematic in your planning, for without this you are extremely unlikely to meet all or any of your goals.

- very motivating, for you can look back and see the progress you have made over weeks and months (and ultimately even years); it will remind you of how hard and well you have trained.

- valuable, because you are constantly reminded of your goals, which helps to focus your training and remind you when it's time to rest.

- informative, for you can see what is working well and less well; you may notice patterns in your training behaviour, and you will even be able to pick up signs of overtraining before they become serious and result in injury or illness.

- helpful in managing your rehabilitation back to fitness should you become injured.
- helpful for your coach, who will know what you are doing and feeling.

The way to make it less of a chore is to design it yourself so it fully meets your needs and can be done in a way that you find interesting (and even enjoyable). In this section, you can examine a sample diary and then decide whether you want to continue to use your current training diary, adapt your current diary, or design and develop a new training diary.

It is divided into two parts:

1. Recording your progress
2. Sample diary pages

If you have never kept a diary before, writing down what you have done in training each day might feel a little strange at first. On the other hand, if you have used a training diary before, it should feel like an old friend.

Recording Your Progress

Before you start a diary, think about how and when you will use it.

- Will you want a diary that holds everything from your personal information (birthdays, special days, meetings) to all your training diary details (seasonal goals and planners, personal bests, weekly plans and logs, daily records and your thoughts)?
- When will you complete it? This might tell you something about the best size and format. Do you want to carry it around with you in your training kit? In your school bag? Leave it by your bed or at your desk?
- Do you like a set format to complete every day, or do you prefer to have an empty page and record what's important?
- Exactly what information will you record?

You will probably want to record some or all of the following:

- Your seasonal (and longer-term) goals
- Your yearly planner
- Your personal profile
- Your shorter-term goals and action plans
- Weekly goals and planners
- Weekly record of training, including personal details such as body weight, resting heart rate (this gives a good indication of training adaptation), sleep patterns and attitude towards training

- Pre-competition strategy sheet
- Competition evaluation sheet
- Competition results

Your weekly record of training is the main part of your diary and should record what training you did (technical, tactical, fitness and mental training) and how you felt. For example, if it was a technique session, make a note of which parts of your technique you worked on, the drills carried out and how well you did. If it was a fitness session, record what you did, as well as times, distances or weight lifted and recovery times. If it was a session conducted outside, record what the conditions were like and how they affected you.

Sample Diary Pages

You are invited to use or adapt the following diary as you think appropriate. You may have to try out different diary formats until you find one that really works for you. Be willing to change it as necessary.

Once you have completed the annual planner, it would be useful to make enough copies for yourself (pinned up in your bedroom), your parent or guardian (pinned up in the kitchen), your coach (pinned up at the club) and your teacher (kept somewhere safe for reference).

Where you have identified hot spots, you need to sit down with your coach, parent or guardian and teacher to sort out how they can help you make the most of the time you have available and what your priorities will be. You will probably find that simply completing the training planner and giving out copies to your coach, teacher and parent or guardian will make them realise what a difficult balancing act you have on your hands.

To help you commit to completing your training diary, try to get into a habit about when you make your diary entries (e.g., just before you go to sleep).

Good luck with your training diary, and may you have all the sporting success you deserve.

Key Points

- Keep a diary to help you plan, monitor and record your progress against your goals.
- Give a copy of your annual planner to your parent or guardian, your coach and your teacher so they can help you prioritise.

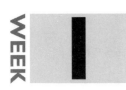

DIARY SHEET

	Competitions	Training	Academic	Social
Mon.				
Tues.				
Wed.				
Thurs.				
Fri.				
Sat.				
Sun.				

DIARY SHEET

	Competitions	Training	Academic	Social
Mon.				
Tues.				
Wed.				
Thurs.				
Fri.				
Sat.				
Sun.				

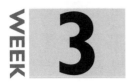
DIARY SHEET

	Competitions	Training	Academic	Social
Mon.				
Tues.				
Wed.				
Thurs.				
Fri.				
Sat.				
Sun.				

DIARY SHEET

	Competitions	Training	Academic	Social
Mon.				
Tues.				
Wed.				
Thurs.				
Fri.				
Sat.				
Sun.				

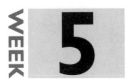

DIARY SHEET

	Competitions	Training	Academic	Social
Mon.				
Tues.				
Wed.				
Thurs.				
Fri.				
Sat.				
Sun.				

DIARY SHEET

	Competitions	Training	Academic	Social
Mon.				
Tues.				
Wed.				
Thurs.				
Fri.				
Sat.				
Sun.				

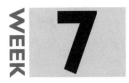

DIARY SHEET

	Competitions	Training	Academic	Social
Mon.				
Tues.				
Wed.				
Thurs.				
Fri.				
Sat.				
Sun.				

DIARY SHEET

	Competitions	Training	Academic	Social
Mon.				
Tues.				
Wed.				
Thurs.				
Fri.				
Sat.				
Sun.				

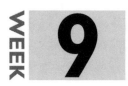

WEEK

DIARY SHEET

	Competitions	Training	Academic	Social
Mon.				
Tues.				
Wed.				
Thurs.				
Fri.				
Sat.				
Sun.				

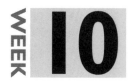

DIARY SHEET

	Competitions	Training	Academic	Social
Mon.				
Tues.				
Wed.				
Thurs.				
Fri.				
Sat.				
Sun.				

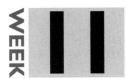

DIARY SHEET

	Competitions	Training	Academic	Social
Mon.				
Tues.				
Wed.				
Thurs.				
Fri.				
Sat.				
Sun.				

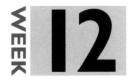

DIARY SHEET

	Competitions	Training	Academic	Social
Mon.				
Tues.				
Wed.				
Thurs.				
Fri.				
Sat.				
Sun.				

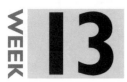

DIARY SHEET

	Competitions	Training	Academic	Social
Mon.				
Tues.				
Wed.				
Thurs.				
Fri.				
Sat.				
Sun.				

DIARY SHEET

	Competitions	Training	Academic	Social
Mon.				
Tues.				
Wed.				
Thurs.				
Fri.				
Sat.				
Sun.				

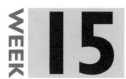

DIARY SHEET

	Competitions	Training	Academic	Social
Mon.				
Tues.				
Wed.				
Thurs.				
Fri.				
Sat.				
Sun.				

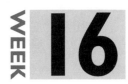

DIARY SHEET

	Competitions	Training	Academic	Social
Mon.				
Tues.				
Wed.				
Thurs.				
Fri.				
Sat.				
Sun.				

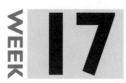

DIARY SHEET

	Competitions	Training	Academic	Social
Mon.				
Tues.				
Wed.				
Thurs.				
Fri.				
Sat.				
Sun.				

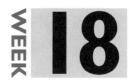

DIARY SHEET

	Competitions	Training	Academic	Social
Mon.				
Tues.				
Wed.				
Thurs.				
Fri.				
Sat.				
Sun.				

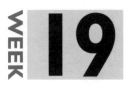

DIARY SHEET

	Competitions	Training	Academic	Social
Mon.				
Tues.				
Wed.				
Thurs.				
Fri.				
Sat.				
Sun.				

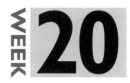

DIARY SHEET

	Competitions	Training	Academic	Social
Mon.				
Tues.				
Wed.				
Thurs.				
Fri.				
Sat.				
Sun.				

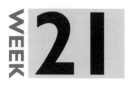

DIARY SHEET

	Competitions	Training	Academic	Social
Mon.				
Tues.				
Wed.				
Thurs.				
Fri.				
Sat.				
Sun.				

DIARY SHEET

	Competitions	Training	Academic	Social
Mon.				
Tues.				
Wed.				
Thurs.				
Fri.				
Sat.				
Sun.				

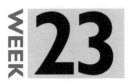

DIARY SHEET

	Competitions	Training	Academic	Social
Mon.				
Tues.				
Wed.				
Thurs.				
Fri.				
Sat.				
Sun.				

DIARY SHEET

	Competitions	Training	Academic	Social
Mon.				
Tues.				
Wed.				
Thurs.				
Fri.				
Sat.				
Sun.				

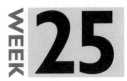

DIARY SHEET

	Competitions	Training	Academic	Social
Mon.				
Tues.				
Wed.				
Thurs.				
Fri.				
Sat.				
Sun.				

DIARY SHEET

	Competitions	Training	Academic	Social
Mon.				
Tues.				
Wed.				
Thurs.				
Fri.				
Sat.				
Sun.				

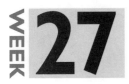

DIARY SHEET

	Competitions	Training	Academic	Social
Mon.				
Tues.				
Wed.				
Thurs.				
Fri.				
Sat.				
Sun.				

DIARY SHEET

	Competitions	Training	Academic	Social
Mon.				
Tues.				
Wed.				
Thurs.				
Fri.				
Sat.				
Sun.				

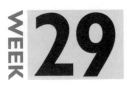

DIARY SHEET

	Competitions	Training	Academic	Social
Mon.				
Tues.				
Wed.				
Thurs.				
Fri.				
Sat.				
Sun.				

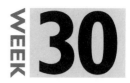

DIARY SHEET

	Competitions	Training	Academic	Social
Mon.				
Tues.				
Wed.				
Thurs.				
Fri.				
Sat.				
Sun.				

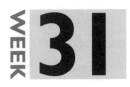

DIARY SHEET

	Competitions	Training	Academic	Social
Mon.				
Tues.				
Wed.				
Thurs.				
Fri.				
Sat.				
Sun.				

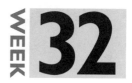
DIARY SHEET

	Competitions	Training	Academic	Social
Mon.				
Tues.				
Wed.				
Thurs.				
Fri.				
Sat.				
Sun.				

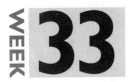

DIARY SHEET

	Competitions	Training	Academic	Social
Mon.				
Tues.				
Wed.				
Thurs.				
Fri.				
Sat.				
Sun.				

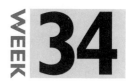

DIARY SHEET

	Competitions	Training	Academic	Social
Mon.				
Tues.				
Wed.				
Thurs.				
Fri.				
Sat.				
Sun.				

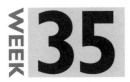

DIARY SHEET

	Competitions	Training	Academic	Social
Mon.				
Tues.				
Wed.				
Thurs.				
Fri.				
Sat.				
Sun.				

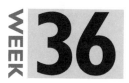
DIARY SHEET

	Competitions	Training	Academic	Social
Mon.				
Tues.				
Wed.				
Thurs.				
Fri.				
Sat.				
Sun.				

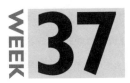

DIARY SHEET

	Competitions	Training	Academic	Social
Mon.				
Tues.				
Wed.				
Thurs.				
Fri.				
Sat.				
Sun.				

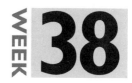

DIARY SHEET

	Competitions	Training	Academic	Social
Mon.				
Tues.				
Wed.				
Thurs.				
Fri.				
Sat.				
Sun.				

DIARY SHEET

	Competitions	Training	Academic	Social
Mon.				
Tues.				
Wed.				
Thurs.				
Fri.				
Sat.				
Sun.				

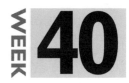

DIARY SHEET

	Competitions	Training	Academic	Social
Mon.				
Tues.				
Wed.				
Thurs.				
Fri.				
Sat.				
Sun.				

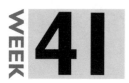

DIARY SHEET

	Competitions	Training	Academic	Social
Mon.				
Tues.				
Wed.				
Thurs.				
Fri.				
Sat.				
Sun.				

DIARY SHEET

	Competitions	Training	Academic	Social
Mon.				
Tues.				
Wed.				
Thurs.				
Fri.				
Sat.				
Sun.				

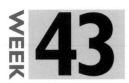

DIARY SHEET

	Competitions	Training	Academic	Social
Mon.				
Tues.				
Wed.				
Thurs.				
Fri.				
Sat.				
Sun.				

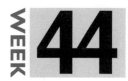

DIARY SHEET

	Competitions	Training	Academic	Social
Mon.				
Tues.				
Wed.				
Thurs.				
Fri.				
Sat.				
Sun.				

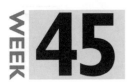
DIARY SHEET

	Competitions	Training	Academic	Social
Mon.				
Tues.				
Wed.				
Thurs.				
Fri.				
Sat.				
Sun.				

DIARY SHEET

	Competitions	Training	Academic	Social
Mon.				
Tues.				
Wed.				
Thurs.				
Fri.				
Sat.				
Sun.				

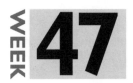

DIARY SHEET

	Competitions	Training	Academic	Social
Mon.				
Tues.				
Wed.				
Thurs.				
Fri.				
Sat.				
Sun.				

DIARY SHEET

	Competitions	Training	Academic	Social
Mon.				
Tues.				
Wed.				
Thurs.				
Fri.				
Sat.				
Sun.				

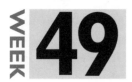

DIARY SHEET

	Competitions	Training	Academic	Social
Mon.				
Tues.				
Wed.				
Thurs.				
Fri.				
Sat.				
Sun.				

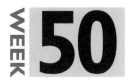

DIARY SHEET

	Competitions	Training	Academic	Social
Mon.				
Tues.				
Wed.				
Thurs.				
Fri.				
Sat.				
Sun.				

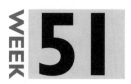

DIARY SHEET

	Competitions	Training	Academic	Social
Mon.				
Tues.				
Wed.				
Thurs.				
Fri.				
Sat.				
Sun.				

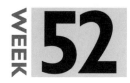

DIARY SHEET

	Competitions	Training	Academic	Social
Mon.				
Tues.				
Wed.				
Thurs.				
Fri.				
Sat.				
Sun.				

ABOUT THE YOUTH SPORT TRUST

The **Youth Sport Trust** is a young, dynamic charity established in 1994 and supported by many of the key names in British sport, such as Sebastian Coe, Sue Barker and Mike Atherton. The Trust believes that physical activity and sport have a key role in the development of all young people. Therefore, the Trust works to build a brighter future for young people in sport.

The Trust's mission is to develop and implement, in close partnership with other organizations, quality physical education (PE) and sport programmes for all young people ages 18 months to 18 years in schools and in the community. In doing so, the YST has teamed up with Human Kinetics as its official publisher, and this is the first of many ongoing projects between the UK's foremost PE trust and the world's premier publisher in physical activity.

The Youth Sport Trust is committed to working with a range of organisations, including schools, universities and sport teams, to provide support to talented and gifted young athletes. *The Young Athlete's Handbook* is compiled from the notes of some of the UK's top coaches and sport experts. These professionals' techniques have been tested at performance camps run by the Youth Sport Trust at Loughborough University.

You'll find
other outstanding
youth sport resources at

www.humankinetics.com

In the U.K. and Europe call

+44 (0) 113 278 1708

Australia 08 8277 1555
Canada 1-800-465-7301
New Zealand 09-523-3462
United States 1-800-747-4457

HUMAN KINETICS
The Premier Publisher for Sports & Fitness